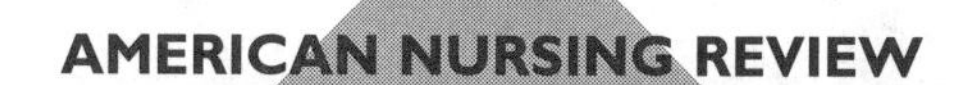

Questions & Answers FOR NCLEX-RN

Second Edition

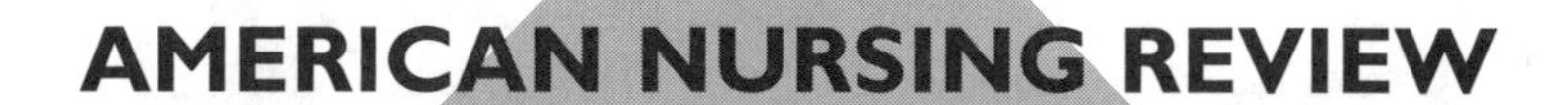

AMERICAN NURSING REVIEW

Questions & Answers FOR NCLEX-RN

Second Edition

Phyllis F. Healy, RN,C, PhD

Kathleen M. Maher, RN, MSN

SPRINGHOUSE CORPORATION ■ SPRINGHOUSE, PENNSYLVANIA

Staff

Vice President
Matthew Cahill

Clinical Director
Judith Schilling McCann, RN, MSN

Art Director
John Hubbard

Managing Editor
David Moreau

Clinical Editor
Collette Bishop Hendler, RN, CCRN

Editors
Karen Diamond, Margaret MacKay Eckman

Copy Editors
Brenna H. Mayer (manager), Priscilla DeWitt, Mary T. Durkin, Stacey A. Follin, Barbara Long, Pamela Wingrod

Designers
Arlene Putterman (associate art director), Lesley Weissman-Cook (book design), Susan Sheridan (project manager), Donna S. Morris

Manufacturing
Deborah Meiris (director), Patricia K. Dorshaw (manager), Otto Mezei

Editorial Assistants
Beverly Lane, Marcia Mills, Liz Schaeffer

Indexer
Manjit K. Sahai

The clinical procedures described and recommended in this publication are based on research and consultation with nursing, medical, and legal authorities. To the best of our knowledge, these procedures reflect currently accepted practice; nevertheless, they cannot be considered absolute and universal recommendations. For individual application, all recommendations must be considered in light of the patient's clinical condition and, before administration of new or infrequently used drugs, in light of the latest package-insert information. The author and the publisher disclaim responsibility for any adverse effects resulting directly or indirectly from the suggested procedures, from any undetected errors, or from the reader's misunderstanding of the text.

Printed in the United States of America.
QARN-020599

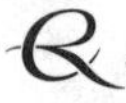 A member of the Reed Elsevier plc group

Library of Congress Cataloging-in-Publication Data
Healy, Phyllis F.
American nursing review: questions and answers for NCLEX-RN / Phyllis F. Healy, Kathleen M. Maher. — 2nd ed.
p. cm.
Includes bibliographical references and index.
1. Practical nursing—Examinations, questions, etc. I. Maher, Kathleen M. II. Title. III. Title: Questions and answers for NCLEX-RN. [DNLM: 1. Nursing, Practical examination questions. WY 18.2 H4345a 1999]
RT62.H43 1999
610.73'06'93076—dc21
DNLM/DLC 98-49377
ISBN 0-87434-983-4 (alk. paper) CIP

CONTENTS

Contributors

American Nursing Review wishes to thank the following people for their contributions:

Exzelia D. Alfred, RN, MA, MEd
Richardean Benjamin, RN, MSN, PhD
Janice Betz, RN, MSN, CS, CNOR
Suzanne C. Beyea, RN, MSN, PhD
Barbara Bloink, RN, MSN
Ruth Brewer, RN, PhD
Ann B. Broussard, RN, MSN
Carolyn Cagle, RN, PhD
Jan Crissinger, RN, ADN
Sandra Czerwinski, RN, MS, CCRN
Barbara Dion, RN, MSN
Catherine Eddy, RN, MSN, CCRN
Susan Everhart, RN, MA, CPNP
Carolyn Fakouri, RN, DNS
Sharon Falkenstern, RN, CRNP, MSN
Eileen Fowles, RN,C, MSN
Sally Friedman, RN, BSN
Patricia Gambill, RN,C, MSN
Laura Gantt, RN, MSN
Michele Gerwick, RN, MSN
Mary Lou Hamilton, RN, MS
Peggy Harris, RN, EdD
Sarah A. Hitchcock, RN, MS, PNP
Rosemary L. Hoffmann, RN, MSN
Brenda Holloway, RN, MSN, CFNP
Mary Lou Holmes, RN, MSN, CS
Karrie S. Ingalsbe, RN, MSN
Helen Jacobson, RN, MSN
Rosalind Kahn, RN, MSN, ARNP
Mary E. Keaveny, RN, MSN
Gloria Kersey-Matusiak, RN, MSN
Jane C. Kinyon, RN, MSN
Linda Kmetz, RN, PhD
Jane Koeckeritz, RN, PhD, ANP
Ruth Lange, RN, BSN
Audrey LaPenta, RN, MA
Elizabeth A. Lorenzi, RN, MSN
Judy W. Maurer, RN, MSN
Carrie A. McCoy, RN, MSN
Dee McGonigle, RN,C, PhD
Karen McGough, RN, MS, ARNP, OCN
Emily McKinney, RN, MSN
Rosemary McLaughlin, RN, MN, CS
Janis A. Metro-Emmert, RN, MSN
Carmella Mikol, RN, MN, CPNP
Aletta L. Moffett, RN, MSN
Barbara A. Moynihan, RN, MN, CS
Carol Muha-Ronneau, RN, MSN
Deborah Nelson, RN, MSN
Mary Pappas, RN, MSN, CANP
Kathy Pickrell, RN, MSN
Reta M. Porter, RN, MSN
Susan Pryor, RN, MN
Larry Purnell, RN, PhD
Joan A. Reider, RN, DNSc
Silvana F. Richardson, RN, PhD
Linda Servidio, RN, MSN
Dianne Siewert, RN, MSN
Marilyn Simons, RN, MSN
Karen Skillings, RN, MSN, ARNP
Koreen Smiley, RN, MSN
Dorothy Woods Smith, RN, PhD
Patricia Solano, RN, BSN
Annette Stacy, RN, MSN
Jeanne Venhaus Stein, RN, MSN
Marian Stewart, RN, MSN
Sharon Strang, RN, MSN
Louise Suit, RN, EdD
Kay I. Swiger, RN,C, MN
Mary Thornton, RN, MS
Lynne Tier, RN, MSN
Elizabeth J. Tipping, RN, MN
Ann B. Tritak, RN, EdD
Linda Ulak, RN, EdD
Loretta Wack, RN, MSN, FNP
Bernadette Walz, RN, MSN
Mary Wessinger, RN,C, MN
Elva J. Winter, RN, PhD, CS
Tamra Young, RN, BSN

PREFACE

Completing the National Council Licensure Examination for Registered Nurses (NCLEX-RN) is the final step in your preparation for nursing practice. Success on this all-important test demands that you develop and follow a carefully constructed plan. Experience proves that a sound nursing education program—combined with a well-designed study program that may include group study or a review course—is the best way to achieve success on the licensure examination.

American Nursing Review: Questions and Answers for NCLEX-RN, Second Edition, provides all the information you need to ensure success on the examination:

- It covers the computerized adaptive test (CAT) format, providing the latest information about the test, its construction, and administration.
- It contains hundreds of thoughtfully crafted questions that follow the latest NCLEX-RN test format. You'll find questions in all four clinical practice areas (mental health, maternal-infant, child, and adult nursing), with such key topics as nutrition, pharmacology, legal issues, and staff management woven through each chapter.
- It provides rationales for the correct answer to each question and also explains why the other options are incorrect. In addition, for each question, the rationale section reveals the applicable phase of the nursing process (NP), client needs category (CN) and client needs subcategory (CNS), cognitive level (CL), and, for the posttest, clinical area (CA).
- It offers a convenient two-column format (questions on the left, answers and rationales on the right) that provides instant feedback, eliminating the need to flip to the back of the book for every correct answer (unlike most other review books).

This Q&A book consists of six chapters, each containing important information to help you prepare properly for the test.

Chapter 1, Understanding NCLEX-RN CAT, provides helpful information on registration, test sites, and schedules. It describes the new CAT format, reviews the main components of the NCLEX-RN test plan, and offers valuable test-taking hints and strategies that will enhance your success during study and on the day of the test.

Chapter 2, Mental Health Nursing, covers the spectrum of mental health and illness, including anorexia nervosa, bipolar disorder, bulimia, child abuse, obsessive-compulsive disorder, organic mental disorder, and voluntary and involuntary admissions.

Chapter 3, Maternal-Infant Nursing, focuses on maternal, fetal, and neonatal well-being, with questions on abruptio placentae, labor induction, placenta previa, pregnancy-induced hypertension, and well-baby care, among other topics.

Chapter 4, Child Nursing, quizzes the reader on such pediatric problems as cleft lip and palate, croup, ear infections, leukemia, and sickle cell anemia.

Chapter 5, Adult Nursing, reviews such topics as acquired immunodeficiency syndrome, Addison's disease, cerebrovascular accident, colorectal cancer, myocardial infarction, and rheumatoid arthritis.

Chapter 6, Posttest, integrates 60 questions of varying difficulty from all four clinical areas, just like the actual examination.

The book concludes with a list of selected references for further investigation of critical issues and an index that enables you to find key topics quickly.

American Nursing Review: Questions and Answers for NCLEX-RN, Second Edition, is the perfect study tool for those planning to take the NCLEX-RN and the perfect instrument for nurses who want to test or review their clinical knowledge. We wish you the best of luck on NCLEX-RN and a rewarding career as a professional RN.

F. William Balkie, RN, MBA, CRNA
President
American Nursing Review

Jenkin V. Williams
Executive Vice President
American Nursing Review

Understanding NCLEX-RN CAT

Anyone who wants to practice as a registered nurse in the United States must be licensed by the nursing licensure authority in the state or territory in which he or she intends to practice. To obtain this license, you must pass the National Council Licensure Examination for Registered Nurses (NCLEX-RN).

Your success on the NCLEX-RN depends on your nursing knowledge base, your study program for the test, your level of confidence, and your familiarity with computerized adaptive testing (CAT). Understandably, you may feel anxious about taking the exam on a computer, especially if you haven't had much practice with one. This chapter provides helpful information about the test, acquaints you with the new computerized format, and gives you effective strategies for passing it.

REGISTRATION, TEST SITES, AND SCHEDULES

Once you have met all eligibility requirements to be a professional nurse, you must apply to take the NCLEX-RN through the board of nursing in the state where you live or plan to work. Shortly after your application is approved, you will receive an "Authorization to Test" from the Educational Testing Service (ETS) Data Center. This authorization will instruct you to make an appointment to take the exam at a Sylvan Technology Center of your choice. More than 200 of these centers are located throughout the United States, with at least one in each state or territory. Each center will have up to 10 computer terminals available for candidates. A proctor will assist you in getting started and will monitor security during the test.

The computerized NCLEX-RN, which lasts a maximum of 5 hours, is offered 15 hours every day, Monday through Saturday, throughout the year (on Sundays only when necessary to meet peak demands). You will take the test no later than 30 days from the day you call to schedule it, so be sure that you are thoroughly prepared when you call. If you are being retested after failing the exam, your test date will be within 45 days of your call. You may reschedule without charge by telephoning the test center at least 3 days before your test date.

COMPUTERIZED ADAPTIVE TESTING

Until recently, the NCLEX-RN had been a paper-and-pencil examination in which candidates had to answer a predetermined number of questions correctly in order to pass. Beginning in April 1994, the format changed to a computerized test in which the candidate must answer enough questions of varying levels of difficulty to demonstrate minimum competence as an entry-level nurse.

The CAT differs from the paper-and-pencil test in other ways. Of course, the most obvious difference is that, instead of sitting at a table with a test book and a pencil, you will sit in front of a computer terminal, interacting with it as you take the NCLEX-RN.

APPEARANCE OF QUESTIONS ON THE COMPUTER SCREEN

Questions on the computerized NCLEX-RN are structured in one of two ways, as shown below. Some questions are based on brief case studies, which appear to the left of the question; others are stand-alone items.

An 18-year-old client is admitted to the hospital with generalized seizures. He is placed on seizure precautions.	Which of the following should the nurse focus on during the initial assessment? 1. Level of excitability 2. Eating of foods high in tyramine 3. Presence of an aura 4. Ridges on the client's fingernails

What would be the priority postoperative goal for a 65-year-old client admitted for a femoropopliteal bypass graft of the left leg?	1. Prevent graft occlusion. 2. Prevent infection at the graft site. 3. Relieve postoperative pain. 4. Maintain adequate fluid and nutrition balance.

The CAT chooses test items based on your response to the previous question; that is, the computer will "adapt" to each answer, correct or incorrect, by selecting a harder or easier item for the next question. For example, at the start of the exam, you'll be given a question of medium-level difficulty. If you answer the question correctly, the computer will then ask a more difficult question. If you answer incorrectly, the computer will ask an easier question.

The test bank contains thousands of questions, each categorized according to the NCLEX-RN test plan and assigned a level of difficulty using a complex statistical formula. Every time you answer a question, the computer searches the test bank for an appropriate next question based on the difficulty of the previous question and the accuracy of your response. This process continues until the computer can determine your competence in all areas of the test plan. Because each test is individualized, the number of questions can range from 75 to 265 (15 of these will be practice questions).

The computerized test begins with brief instructions on using the computer and then provides a short practice session. Previous computer experience is not necessary. You will use only two keys on the keyboard: the *space bar* and the *enter key*. All other keys will be nonfunctioning. You will use the space bar to move the cursor among four possible options and press the enter key to record your answer. The computer will then ask you to confirm your choice by pressing the enter key a second time. This ensures that you do not select an answer unintentionally.

One question at a time will appear on the computer screen, shown in one of two formats (see *Appearance of questions on the computer screen*).

After carefully reading the question, press the space bar to move among the four possible options. Analyze each choice and then select the one that best answers the question. Press the enter key twice to record your choice. You must answer every question until the test ends; unlike the paper-and-pencil testing method, the computer will not allow you to skip an item or go back to a previous question.

The test center will transmit your results electronically to ETS. Your state board will notify you of the results in 4 to 6 weeks. No test results are released over the telephone.

NCLEX-RN TEST PLAN

All questions on the computerized NCLEX-RN adhere to a test plan, or blueprint, that organizes questions according to the *client needs* framework. You will also find questions on concepts fundamental to nursing practice integrated throughout the exam.

Client Needs

The client needs framework is the foundation for the examination. This framework offers a basic structure for categorizing nursing behaviors and skills across all clinical areas and in all client settings.

The framework includes four main client needs categories, each with subcategories that further define specific nursing responsibilities. Each item on the test is coded for a client needs subcategory. A specific percentage of questions on the NCLEX-RN comes from each of the subcategories; the percentages are determined every 3 years by a job analysis of entry-level nurses. The four main categories, subcategories and their descriptions, and the percentage of questions from each are listed below, according to the National Council of State Boards of Nursing's detailed test plan for NCLEX-RN.

1. Safe, effective care environment

- *Management of care:* The nurse provides integrated, cost-effective care to clients by coordinating, supervising, and/or collaborating with members of the multidisciplinary health care team. (7% to 13%)
- *Safety and infection control:* The nurse protects clients and health care personnel from environmental hazards. (5% to 11%)

2. Health promotion and maintenance

- *Growth and development through the life span:* The nurse assists clients and their significant others through the normal expected stages of growth and development from conception through advanced old age. (7% to 13%)
- *Prevention and early detection of disease:* The nurse manages and provides care for clients in need of prevention and early detection of health problems. (5% to 11%)

3. Psychosocial integrity

- *Coping and adaptation:* The nurse promotes the ability of clients to cope with, adapt to, and/or problem solve situations related to illnesses or stressful events. (5% to 11%)
- *Psychosocial adaptation:* The nurse manages and provides care for clients with acute or chronic mental illnesses. (5% to 11%)

4. Physiological integrity

- *Basic care and comfort:* The nurse provides comfort and assistance in the performance of activities of daily living. (7% to 13%)
- *Pharmacological and parenteral therapies:* The nurse manages and provides care related to the administration of medications and parenteral therapies. (5% to 11%)
- *Reduction of risk potential:* The nurse provides care that reduces the likelihood that clients will develop complications or health problems related to existing conditions, treatments, or procedures. (12% to 18%)
- *Physiological adaptation:* The nurse manages and provides care to clients with acute, chronic, or life-threatening physical health conditions. (12% to 18%)

Fundamental Concepts

The NCLEX-RN also tests several concepts and processes basic to nursing practice. They include nursing process, caring, communication, cultural awareness, documentation, self-care, and teaching and learning. No specific percentage of questions is assigned to these concepts; they appear throughout the exam.

PREPARING FOR THE EXAMINATION

Proper preparation for the exam involves thorough study and careful planning before the test and mastery of test-taking strategies that you can use during the test. The following tips will help ensure your success on the computerized NCLEX-RN.

Study Thoroughly

- Become well versed in all of the topics that the exam is likely to cover, and answer as many practice questions as you can. After answering the questions in each clinical area of this book, take the sample test in Chapter 6, which will ensure your exposure to all areas of the test plan.
- Become familiar with all parts of a test question (see *Parts of a test question,* page 4).
- Supplement this book with other resources, such as *American Nursing Review for NCLEX-RN,* a complete study guide for the test.

PARTS OF A TEST QUESTION

Multiple-choice questions on the NCLEX-RN are constructed according to strict psychometric standards. As shown below, each question has a stem and four options: a key (correct answer) and three distractors (incorrect answers). A brief case study may precede the question.

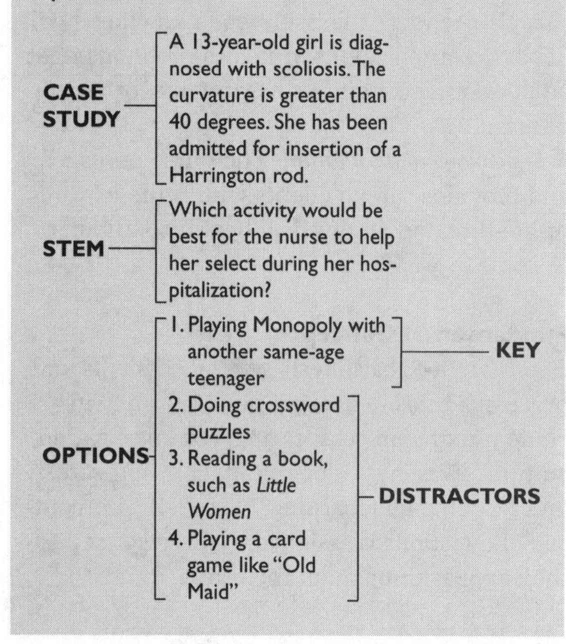

■ Take a review course or organize a study group with others planning to take the exam.
■ Ask a nursing instructor or colleague for help or clarification if you encounter material that is unfamiliar or difficult to understand.

Plan Carefully

■ Schedule your examination at a test site near your residence, if possible, so that you can familiarize yourself with parking facilities and travel time before the test date.
■ If you must travel a lengthy distance and stay overnight, make hotel arrangements well in advance of the test date to ensure that you have a convenient place to stay.
■ Schedule your examination for the time of day that coincides with your peak performance. Some people work best in the early morning; others, in late afternoon or early evening.
■ Get a good night's sleep the night before the test. Staying up late to do last-minute cramming will probably hurt rather than help your performance.
■ Eat a nutritious breakfast on the day of the test.
■ Wear layered clothing so that you can easily adapt to the room temperature at the test center.
■ Keep your admission ticket and identification where you can easily retrieve them when you leave for the test site. You must present your "Authorization to Test" from the ETS Data Center and two forms of identification with your signature, including one photo ID. Without them, you will not be permitted to take the test.
■ Try to avoid last-minute anxiety that could sap your energy or disturb your concentration. Although mild anxiety is normal and can actually heighten your awareness, too much anxiety can impair your performance. If test anxiety has been a problem in the past, practice relaxation techniques (such as guided imagery) as you study, and be ready to use them during the actual test.

Apply Test-Taking Strategies

■ Read case studies carefully. They contain information that you will need to answer the question correctly.
■ Pay special attention to such words as *best, most, first,* and *not* when reading the stem of the question. These words (which may be italicized, capitalized, or otherwise highlighted in some way) usually provide clues to the correct response. For example, consider the question, "What should the nurse do *first?*" All of the listed options may be appropriate nursing actions for the given circumstances, but only one action can take top priority.
■ Try to predict the correct answer as you read the stem of the question. If your predicted answer is among the four options, it is probably the correct response.
■ Read each question and all options carefully before making your selection.
■ Reread two options that seem equally correct; there must be some difference between them. Also reread the stem. You may notice something that you missed before that will aid in your selection. If you still are unsure, make an

educated guess. The computer will not allow you to skip a question.

■ Remain calm if a question focuses on an unfamiliar topic. Try to recall clients who have had problems similar to those in the question. Determine the nursing principles involved in your former clients' care and how they may apply to the test question. This may help you eliminate some options and increase your chances of selecting the right answer.

■ Take the necessary time for each question without spending excessive time on any one item. You will have up to 5 hours to take the test. Pace yourself accordingly.

■ Pay no attention to other candidates or the time they need to complete their tests. Because each test is individualized, some tests contain more questions than others.

■ Take advantage of breaks during the test to give your mind and body a needed rest. The first mandatory break is given after 2 hours of testing and lasts 10 minutes. Candidates may take an optional break 90 minutes after testing resumes. If you tend to get hungry, bring a small snack with you to eat during the breaks. Do some stretching exercises, too, during breaks to help you relax.

Developing and following an organized study plan will provide the best assurance that you are fully prepared to succeed on the NCLEX-RN. Approach the test with confidence. Good luck, and congratulations on choosing nursing as a career.

Mental Health Nursing

1 A 58-year-old client on a mental health unit has lost control, despite having been properly medicated, and is threatening to harm himself and others. He has been placed in four-point restraints. Which nursing measure should be taken next?

☐ 1. Release one restraint every 15 minutes.
☐ 2. Have a staff member stay with the client at all times.
☐ 3. Leave the client alone to reduce his sensory stimulation and allow him to regain control.
☐ 4. Restrict fluids until the restraint period is over.

CORRECT ANSWER: 2
Such a client needs sensory stimulation and should never be left alone (although the nurse should maintain the client's privacy). Option 1: Restraints are removed for 5 minutes at least every 2 hours. Option 3: A client in restraints should have someone with him at all times. Option 4: Fluids are offered, and the client is given food at mealtime.

NP: Implementation
CN: Safe, effective care environment
CNS: Safety and infection control
CL: Application

---

2 Which nursing assessment has priority while a client's extremities are restrained?

☐ 1. Measuring urine output
☐ 2. Checking circulation in extremities
☐ 3. Assessing pupillary responses
☐ 4. Noting respiratory pattern

CORRECT ANSWER: 2
The nurse must check extremities for signs of circulatory impairment. Option 1 is not crucial; the client may void into a urinal as necessary. Option 3 is not relevant to the situation. Option 4: Although the nurse should check vital signs every 15 minutes for 1 hour, assessment for circulation takes priority.

NP: Assessment
CN: Safe, effective care environment
CNS: Safety and infection control
CL: Application

3 A psychiatric client who was voluntarily admitted now wishes to be discharged from the hospital, against medical advice. What is the most important assessment the nurse should make of the client?

☐ 1. Ability to care for self
☐ 2. Degree of danger to self and others
☐ 3. Level of psychosis
☐ 4. Intended compliance with aftercare

CORRECT ANSWER: 2

A voluntary client who poses a danger to self or others may be denied permission to leave the hospital. Options 1, 3, and 4 are important assessments, but the client's danger to self or others takes priority.

NP: Assessment
CN: Safe, effective care environment
CNS: Management of care
CL: Application

---

4 The nurse should determine that restraints are no longer needed when the client does which of the following?

☐ 1. Falls asleep
☐ 2. Ceases verbalizing threats
☐ 3. Is calm verbally and nonverbally
☐ 4. Expresses being OK

CORRECT ANSWER: 3

The nurse should look for consistency in subjective and objective data. Options 1, 2, and 4 may indicate that restraints are no longer needed, but the nurse needs more data than any one of these options provides.

NP: Evaluation
CN: Safe, effective care environment
CNS: Safety and infection control
CL: Application

---

5 A client on an inpatient psychiatric unit at a community mental health center is pacing up and down the hallway. The client has a history of aggression. Which of the following is the nurse's best response when approaching the client?

☐ 1. "If you can't relax, you could go to your room."
☐ 2. "Would you like your antianxiety medication now?"
☐ 3. "You're pacing. What's going on?"
☐ 4. "Let's go play a game of pool."

CORRECT ANSWER: 3

This acknowledges the client's behavior and explores his feelings. Options 1 and 2 assume that the client is anxious, which may be a projection on the nurse's part, considering the client's history of aggression. Option 4 ignores what might be going on with the client.

NP: Implementation
CN: Psychosocial integrity
CNS: Psychosocial adaptation
CL: Analysis

6 A 37-year-old male with a history of schizophrenia is having auditory hallucinations. The physician orders 200 mg of haloperidol (Haldol) orally or I.M. every 4 hours as needed. What is the nurse's best action?

☐ 1. Administer the haloperidol orally if the client agrees to take it.
☐ 2. Call the physician to clarify whether the haloperidol should be given orally or I.M.
☐ 3. Call the physician to clarify the order, because the dosage is too high.
☐ 4. Withhold haloperidol because it may cause hallucinations.

CORRECT ANSWER: 3
The dosage is too high (normal dosage ranges from 5 to 100 mg daily). Options 1 and 2 could cause an overdose. Option 4 is incorrect because haloperidol helps with symptoms of hallucinations.
NP: Implementation
CN: Physiological integrity
CNS: Pharmacological and parenteral therapies
CL: Application

---

7 An inpatient psychiatric client suddenly becomes loud and visibly anxious. What is the best action for the nurse to take?

☐ 1. Summon help and escort the client to his room.
☐ 2. Face the client squarely and say, "You must be quiet."
☐ 3. Say, "Calm down; you're safe here."
☐ 4. Say, "Let's go talk in your room."

CORRECT ANSWER: 4
This acknowledges that the client is important to the nurse and preserves the client's dignity with minimal restriction. Option 1: The client does not need to be escorted to his room at this point; he has not yet been given a chance to go on his own. The nurse should use the least restrictive form of treatment at all times. Option 2: Facing off with the client and demanding quiet is challenging. Option 3 is a placating response, which will likely increase the client's anxiety.
NP: Implementation
CN: Psychosocial integrity
CNS: Psychosocial adaptation
CL: Analysis

---

8 A voluntary client on an inpatient psychiatric unit has a history of auditory hallucinations and self-aggression. The nurse is talking with the client when the client suddenly jumps up and says, to no one in particular, "Get away from me." Which is the nurse's best response?

☐ 1. Escort the client to the client's room.
☐ 2. Say, "I won't let them harm you."
☐ 3. Sit there quietly until the client becomes calm.
☐ 4. Ask, "Who are you talking to?"

CORRECT ANSWER: 4
This question aims to clarify the client's remark. Option 1 ignores what the client said and violates the client's right to the least restrictive environment. Option 2 assumes that the client is hallucinating. Option 3 fails to address what the client said.
NP: Implementation
CN: Psychosocial integrity
CNS: Psychosocial adaptation
CL: Analysis

9 A 35-year-old voluntary client suddenly begins yelling, throws a chair, and exhibits extreme agitation. Which of the following would be most important for the nurse to consider when planning an intervention?

☐ 1. Because the client is a voluntary admission, restraints cannot be used.
☐ 2. The family must be called for permission to restrain the client.
☐ 3. Restraint should be used as a last resort.
☐ 4. Restraint cannot be initiated until the physician is called.

CORRECT ANSWER: 3
Restraint should always be used as a last resort, with the least restrictive measures used first. Option 1: The criteria for restraint involve danger to self or others and do not exclude voluntary clients in emergencies. Option 2: Unless a family member is a guardian, calling the family violates the client's confidentiality. Option 4: In an emergency, the nurse may restrain a client before calling the physician.

NP: Planning
CN: Safe, effective care environment
CNS: Safety and infection control
CL: Application

---

10 Before forcing a client to take a medication, the nurse should give priority to which of the following?

☐ 1. The client's danger to self or others
☐ 2. What the "voices" are saying to the client
☐ 3. Whether the client's admission was voluntary or involuntary
☐ 4. The client's insight into the illness

CORRECT ANSWER: 1
Client rights prohibit the forcing of medication unless the client poses a danger to self or others. If the client is judged incompetent, the guardian or court must approve the forced medication. Options 2, 3, and 4 overrule the client's basic rights.

NP: Assessment
CN: Safe, effective care environment
CNS: Management of care
CL: Application

---

11 A client was admitted to the hospital 2 days ago for disrupting a town meeting, shouting religious delusions, and fighting with police. The client now refuses to take prescribed haloperidol (Haldol), saying, "I don't want it." What is the nurse's best response?

☐ 1. "It will help you feel better."
☐ 2. "You must take it or get an injection."
☐ 3. "What are you afraid of?"
☐ 4. "You sound concerned."

CORRECT ANSWER: 4
The nurse's open-ended response encourages exploration. Option 1 is placating the client. Option 2 is threatening or, at least, too restrictive, because the client has not exhibited dangerous behavior. Option 3 assumes that the client is afraid.

NP: Implementation
CN: Psychosocial integrity
CNS: Psychosocial adaptation
CL: Application

12 A client has been prescribed 75 mg of amitriptyline (Elavil) at bedtime and 15 mg of phenelzine (Nardil) three times a day. Which nursing action takes priority?

☐ 1. Teach the client about the adverse effects.
☐ 2. Call the physician and question the order.
☐ 3. Institute dietary restrictions.
☐ 4. Take baseline vital signs.

CORRECT ANSWER: 2
Administering amitriptyline (a tricyclic antidepressant) and phenelzine (a monoamine oxidase [MAO] inhibitor) together could cause hypertension, tachycardia, or a potentially fatal reaction; the nurse should call the physician to check the order. Options 1, 3, and 4 are important nursing actions, but they do not take priority over calling the physician.
NP: Implementation
CN: Physiological integrity
CNS: Pharmacological and parenteral therapies
CL: Application

---

13 A client on an inpatient psychiatric unit has been taking a tricyclic antidepressant without satisfactory results, so the physician changes to an MAO inhibitor. In evaluating the physician's order, the nurse must first be sure of which of the following?

☐ 1. Adequate time has elapsed between discontinuing the first medication and beginning the second.
☐ 2. The MAO inhibitor is begun at the same dosage as the tricyclic antidepressant.
☐ 3. The client is not suicidal.
☐ 4. The client is not allergic to cheese.

CORRECT ANSWER: 1
Administering these two medications within a short time frame increases the risk of hypertension and hyperpyrexia. Option 2: Dosages of these medications can vary widely. Options 3 and 4 are irrelevant to the choice of drug or timing of administration.
NP: Analysis
CN: Physiological integrity
CNS: Pharmacological and parenteral therapies
CL: Analysis

---

14 A client reports no improvement in mood since beginning a regimen of 15 mg of tranylcypromine (Parnate) twice a day 1 week ago. Which of the following is the best nursing action?

☐ 1. Say to the client, "The medication may need up to 4 weeks to take effect."
☐ 2. Say to the client, "You should feel the effects any day now."
☐ 3. Consult with the physician about a dosage adjustment.
☐ 4. Consult with the physician about a change of medication.

CORRECT ANSWER: 1
MAO inhibitors, such as tranylcypromine, may take up to 4 weeks before improving the client's mood. Option 2 is a vague promise that may create unrealistic expectations in the client. Options 3 and 4 are premature.
NP: Implementation
CN: Physiological integrity
CNS: Pharmacological and parenteral therapies
CL: Application

15 A client who has been hospitalized with depression is about to be discharged with a prescription of phenelzine (Nardil). In planning for discharge, the nurse should have a teaching plan that emphasizes which of the following?

☐ 1. Get adequate rest.
☐ 2. Avoid smoking.
☐ 3. Avoid red wine.
☐ 4. Take the drug with food or milk.

CORRECT ANSWER: 3
A client taking phenelzine (an MAO inhibitor) must avoid foods that contain tyramine (such as red wine) to prevent a hypertensive or hyperpyretic crisis. Options 1 and 2 are healthy behaviors to reinforce, but they do not relate directly to phenelzine. Option 4 may be recommended if the medication causes GI distress, but it is secondary to teaching about the food restrictions.

NP: Implementation
CN: Physiological integrity
CNS: Pharmacological and parenteral therapies
CL: Application

---

16 The physician prescribes an MAO inhibitor for a client. Which of the following nursing diagnostic categories would be most appropriate to focus on during client teaching?

☐ 1. Risk for injury
☐ 2. Altered thought processes
☐ 3. Fluid volume deficit
☐ 4. Sleep pattern disturbance

CORRECT ANSWER: 1
Because an MAO inhibitor can cause hypotension, the client must be given precautions related to driving. Options 2 and 4 are possible but not likely, and they have lower priority than client safety. Option 3 is incorrect because a fluid volume excess is more likely than a deficit.

NP: Analysis
CN: Physiological integrity
CNS: Pharmacological and parenteral therapies
CL: Application

---

17 A nurse is teaching clients in an outpatient clinic about MAO inhibitors. The nurse would best evaluate the clients' understanding of how their medications work by noting which of the following?

☐ 1. Food selections
☐ 2. Fluid intake
☐ 3. Potential for self-harm
☐ 4. Level of anxiety

CORRECT ANSWER: 1
A client taking an MAO inhibitor must avoid tyramine-rich foods to prevent a hypertensive or hyperpyretic crisis. Options 2, 3, and 4 are important assessment areas, but they do not relate directly to the clients' understanding of medications.

NP: Evaluation
CN: Physiological integrity
CNS: Pharmacological and parenteral therapies
CL: Application

18 A hospitalized client taking 30 mg of tranylcypromine (Parnate) twice a day complains of a stiff neck and headache. What is the nurse's best action?

☐ 1. Note the complaints as usual adverse effects.
☐ 2. Withhold the next dose of medication.
☐ 3. Administer an analgesic, as needed and as prescribed.
☐ 4. Help the client relax.

CORRECT ANSWER: 2
A stiff neck and headache may be prodromal symptoms of hypertensive crisis. Option 1: Rather than dismiss the symptoms, the nurse should continue to assess them and consult the physician. Options 3 and 4 would be appropriate measures for a tension headache.
NP: Implementation
CN: Physiological integrity
CNS: Pharmacological and parenteral therapies
CL: Analysis

---

19 A client avoids leaving home to shop for groceries or complete other errands. At times, the client feels "crazy" because of her fear. The client seeks out her neighbor, a nurse, for help. The nurse's assessment is phobic reaction. Which of the following statements about a phobia is true?

☐ 1. The condition is a persistent, intrusive image that seems senseless to the person.
☐ 2. It is important not to force the person to face the phobic object or situation.
☐ 3. The phobic condition can be cured by hypnosis.
☐ 4. It is necessary to agree with the client's assessment that the phobia is silly.

CORRECT ANSWER: 2
Forcing can provoke panic in the client; gradual desensitization is more successful. Option 1 defines an obsession. Option 3 (hypnosis) is used to help identify sources of anxiety responsible for amnesia and fugue and in establishing contact with a client who has multiple-personality disorder. Option 4 fails to acknowledge that the phobia serves a purpose for the person and thus inhibits insight.
NP: Implementation
CN: Psychosocial integrity
CNS: Psychosocial adaptation
CL: Comprehension

---

20 A 76-year-old widowed mother of six is admitted to a long-term care facility with a diagnosis of organic mental disorder. Which of the following approaches would be most helpful for the nurse in meeting the client's needs?

☐ 1. Make sure the client completes tasks that she begins.
☐ 2. Maintain a gentle approach that does not set limits.
☐ 3. Give the client alternative choices in making decisions.
☐ 4. Simplify the environment as much as possible.

CORRECT ANSWER: 4
This helps maintain the client's orientation and prevents further confusion from overstimulation. Options 1 and 3 may confuse a client with organic mental disorder, who typically cannot make decisions and is easily distracted. Option 2 also is incorrect; it is necessary for all staff members to consistently set limits to lower anxiety and increase orientation.
NP: Implementation
CN: Psychosocial integrity
CNS: Psychosocial adaptation
CL: Application

21 Which of the following snacks would be best for a client with anorexia nervosa who requires a high-protein, high-calorie diet?

☐ 1. Chicken soup and crackers
☐ 2. Doughnut and orange juice
☐ 3. Egg salad and peanuts
☐ 4. Cashews and strawberries

CORRECT ANSWER: 3

Egg salad and peanuts are high in protein and calories. Chicken soup and crackers (Option 1) and strawberries (Option 4) are low-protein, low-calorie foods. A doughnut and orange juice (Option 2) are low in protein.

NP: Implementation
CN: Physiological integrity
CNS: Basic care and comfort
CL: Application

---

22 Which is the most appropriate nursing diagnosis for a client exhibiting obsessive-compulsive behavior?

☐ 1. Ineffective individual coping
☐ 2. Altered nutrition: less than body requirements
☐ 3. Altered nutrition: more than body requirements
☐ 4. Altered family processes

CORRECT ANSWER: 1

The client's coping skills are ineffective when anxiety increases. Options 2, 3, and 4 do not correspond to the observed behavior.

NP: Assessment
CN: Psychosocial integrity
CNS: Psychosocial adaptation
CL: Application

---

23 A 28-year-old accountant is admitted to the neurologic unit after a sudden onset of blindness the day before an important project is due for her boss. After preliminary evaluation and testing yields no positive findings, the physician's initial reaction is that the client may be demonstrating which defense mechanism?

☐ 1. Repression
☐ 2. Transference
☐ 3. Reaction formation
☐ 4. Conversion

CORRECT ANSWER: 4

A person can convert unbearable feelings into a physical symptom with no organic cause. This defense mechanism usually manifests itself near the time of a traumatic or conflict-producing event. The symptom commonly provides attention or a means of escaping the conflict. Option 1 is a defense mechanism in which a person unconsciously keeps unwanted feelings from entering awareness. Option 2 involves the projection of feelings, thoughts, and wishes (positive or negative) onto someone, usually a therapist, who represents a figure from the person's past. Option 3 is a means of alleviating unresolved conflicts between feelings or impulses by reinforcing one feeling and repressing another, thereby disguising the true feelings from the self.

NP: Assessment
CN: Psychosocial integrity
CNS: Coping and adaptation
CL: Analysis

24 A client with bipolar disorder, manic phase, who usually dresses conservatively, appears at breakfast with brightly colored cheeks, wearing a miniskirt, sheer blouse, and designer boots. Which of the following actions should the nurse take to deal with the client's attire?

☐ 1. Redirect the client to her room, and help her put on her more customary clothing.
☐ 2. Allow her the freedom to wear what she prefers for now.
☐ 3. Remind the client of the dress code and the consequences of violation.
☐ 4. Tell the client what to wear, and advise her that she has lost the privilege of choosing her wardrobe.

CORRECT ANSWER: 1

The nurse must protect the client from actions that will cause embarrassment when her condition improves. Option 2 does not remove the client from the embarrassing situation. Options 3 and 4 offer chastisement rather than guidance and support.

NP: Implementation
CN: Psychosocial integrity
CNS: Psychosocial adaptation
CL: Application

---

25 What is the most effective intervention for handling a client with an antisocial personality?

☐ 1. Reason with the client.
☐ 2. Set limits with the client.
☐ 3. Ignore the client.
☐ 4. Agree with the client.

CORRECT ANSWER: 2

Limits must be maintained by all staff members and reinforced with restrictions when rules are broken. Options 1, 3, and 4 do not modify the unwanted behavior.

NP: Implementation
CN: Psychosocial integrity
CNS: Psychosocial adaptation
CL: Application

---

26 A client on the nursing unit, charged with child abuse, does not speak to the staff when approached. What is the nurse's best response to this client?

☐ 1. "If you need me, I will be in the nurses' station."
☐ 2. "You need to come to grips with what has happened."
☐ 3. "Not speaking to the staff won't help your situation."
☐ 4. "Admission to a psychiatric unit can be very difficult."

CORRECT ANSWER: 4

This helps the client realize he is having difficulty, without asking direct questions or focusing on specific behavior. Option 1 constitutes avoidance. Option 2 negates the client's feelings. Option 3 focuses on a specific behavior and does not convey sensitivity or caring.

NP: Implementation
CN: Psychosocial integrity
CNS: Coping and adaptation
CL: Application

27 After refusing to eat for 4 days, a 17-year-old college freshman is referred to the inpatient eating disorders unit of a general hospital. Her affect is flat, her eyes downcast, her long blonde hair dull and limp. Her clothes hang loosely on her body, and she appears sullen and frightened. Her weight on admission is 89 lb (41 kg); her normal weight is 114 lb (52 kg). Which of the following assessments would best enable the nurse to develop a specific nursing diagnosis?

☐ 1. Family history, including genograms
☐ 2. Psychiatric history, including all hospital admissions
☐ 3. Cardiac and respiratory history
☐ 4. Weight loss history and general condition of skin, hair, and nails

CORRECT ANSWER: 4

This will help the nurse formulate a nursing diagnosis that addresses the self-control and compliance needed to regain nutritional requirements. Other important areas to assess include nausea, vomiting, edema, and excretory functions. Options 1, 2, and 3 may yield useful data, but they are not as critical at this early stage.

NP: Assessment
CN: Psychosocial integrity
CNS: Psychosocial adaptation
CL: Analysis

---

28 A client is admitted for a suspected eating disorder. Which of the following statements would indicate that the client may be suffering from anorexia nervosa?

☐ 1. "I've gained 3 pounds in the last month."
☐ 2. "I eat loads of spinach and yellow vegetables each day."
☐ 3. "I'm a perfectionist, and I work hard to get A's."
☐ 4. "I binge frequently in the morning and feel fat."

CORRECT ANSWER: 3

Typically, the anorexic client works hard to achieve perfection and loses the ability to accept help. Option 1 refers to weight gain, which may indicate bulimia. Option 2 is atypical of anorexic clients, who have an intense fear of becoming obese and compulsively resist any attempts at eating. Binge eating (Option 4) is characteristic of bulimia (although bulimics tend to binge more frequently in the evening, and "feeling fat" is characteristic of anorexia).

NP: Assessment
CN: Psychosocial integrity
CNS: Psychosocial adaptation
CL: Analysis

---

29 Which of the following nursing interventions would be included in the care of a client with anorexia nervosa as therapy progresses?

☐ 1. Let the client eat alone to avoid embarrassment.
☐ 2. Weigh the client once a week in the same clothing.
☐ 3. Monitor the client for self-destructive tendencies.
☐ 4. Praise the client for "looking better," and remind the client that she is not "too fat."

CORRECT ANSWER: 3

Self-starvation is life-threatening; the client should be monitored for self-destructive tendencies. Option 1: The nurse must stay with the client during meals to ensure that food is being eaten. Option 2: The client should be weighed three times daily in light clothing to ensure accuracy. Option 4: This response could signal a power struggle with the client and the nurse's unconscious means of exerting control.

NP: Implementation
CN: Psychosocial integrity
CNS: Psychosocial adaptation
CL: Application

30 A client with a personality disorder exhibits manipulative behavior. Care planning for this client should include which of the following?

- ☐ 1. Freedom to do as the client chooses when behavior improves
- ☐ 2. Limitations per unit rules without restrictions for broken rules
- ☐ 3. Reasonable expectations with varying limits
- ☐ 4. Verbal reinforcement when the client functions within established limits

CORRECT ANSWER: 4
This encourages the client to follow unit rules. Options 1, 2, and 3 are inconsistent with changing manipulative behavior.
NP: Planning
CN: Psychosocial integrity
CNS: Psychosocial adaptation
CL: Application

---

31 A 40-year-old woman is brought to the hospital by her husband, who states that she has refused to eat or to get out of bed for 2 days. The woman says that she is tired all the time and does not feel up to going to work. Her admitting diagnosis is major depression. Which question would be most appropriate for the admitting nurse to ask?

- ☐ 1. "What has been troubling you?"
- ☐ 2. "Why do you dislike yourself?"
- ☐ 3. "How do you feel about your life?"
- ☐ 4. "What can we do to help?"

CORRECT ANSWER: 3
The nurse must base nursing interventions on a client's perceived problems and feelings. Option 1 asks the client to draw a conclusion, which she may have difficulty doing at this time. Option 2 places the client in a defensive position. Option 4 is beyond the scope of the client's present abilities; she would probably rather have the nurse tell her how she can help herself.
NP: Implementation
CN: Psychosocial integrity
CNS: Psychosocial adaptation
CL: Application

---

32 A 24-year-old secretary is transferred to your psychiatric unit. Her husband says that she has been overeating and that she vomits soon after she eats. Her weight stays about the same, at 96 lb (44 kg). In planning care for the client, the nurse should anticipate which medical diagnosis?

- ☐ 1. Anorexia nervosa
- ☐ 2. Bulimia
- ☐ 3. Klein-Levin syndrome
- ☐ 4. Dysthymia

CORRECT ANSWER: 2
The client exhibits the binging and purging typical of bulimia. Anorexia nervosa (Option 1) involves severe weight loss. Klein-Levin syndrome (Option 3) includes symptoms of a disturbed eating behavior, but the condition is not characterized by the client's excessive concern with body shape and weight. Dysthymia (Option 4) is a type of depression.
NP: Planning
CN: Psychosocial integrity
CNS: Psychosocial adaptation
CL: Application

33 For a client with bulimia, which assessment is least important in the plan of care?

- ☐ 1. Observe the client after eating for 1 hour.
- ☐ 2. Note the client's intake.
- ☐ 3. Note changes in appetite.
- ☐ 4. Note changes in respiratory rate.

CORRECT ANSWER: 4
Respiratory rate usually is not affected by bulimia. Option 1 is important because it is the time that she is likely to vomit. Option 2 and 3 are important factors to monitor in bulimia or any other eating disorder.
NP: Planning
CN: Physiological integrity
CNS: Basic care and comfort
CL: Application

---

34 A client with personality disorder gets along poorly with the immediate family. The client's manipulative behavior most likely shows a failure to develop which of the following?

- ☐ 1. Intimate relationships
- ☐ 2. Trust
- ☐ 3. Industry
- ☐ 4. Feelings of guilt

CORRECT ANSWER: 2
Manipulative behavior arises from a lack of trust. The client cannot develop trust in others when he does not trust his own feelings. Options 1, 3, and 4 cannot be accomplished until trust is established.
NP: Assessment
CN: Psychosocial integrity
CNS: Coping and adaptation
CL: Application

---

35 A 32-year-old client is admitted to the unit. She states, "I am a well-known, wealthy designer," and begins to order the nurses to prepare her bath while she orders her tray and telephones her colleagues. Her husband states that she is too busy to eat and sleep and is losing weight. Her admitting diagnosis is bipolar disorder, manic phase. Which of the following should the nurse plan for?

- ☐ 1. Erratic and unpredictable behavior if challenged
- ☐ 2. Boredom and the need for minute-to-minute activities
- ☐ 3. Rapid mood changes from elation to depression
- ☐ 4. One-to-one treatment to occupy the client's time

CORRECT ANSWER: 1
Bipolar clients are often unpredictable, with angry outbursts. Options 2 and 4: The unit itself, with its regularly scheduled activities, may provide too much stimulation for the manic client. Option 3: The course of illness would not be expected to move rapidly through the manic-depressive-manic cycle, although the client should be observed for signs of depression.
NP: Planning
CN: Psychosocial integrity
CNS: Psychosocial adaptation
CL: Application

36 A 32-year-old lawyer is admitted to the neurologic unit with a sudden onset of blindness the night before an important case is scheduled to go to trial. Tests reveal no physical findings. Which of the following best analyzes the client's anxiety?

☐ 1. It is diffuse and free floating.
☐ 2. It is consciously experienced.
☐ 3. It is localized and relieved by the blindness.
☐ 4. It is projected onto the environment.

CORRECT ANSWER: 3
Anxiety is relieved by keeping an internal need or conflict out of conscious awareness. The sudden onset of blindness without physiologic basis impairs normal activity and may promote the development of a chronic sick role. The anxiety-provoking impulse (the trial) is converted unconsciously into a functional symptom. Options 1, 2, and 4 do not accurately describe the client's anxiety.

NP: Assessment
CN: Psychosocial integrity
CNS: Coping and adaptation
CL: Analysis

---

37 A 50-year-old client has been admitted for psychological testing after having been charged with physical abuse of a 7-year-old child. The client refuses to come to the dayroom, saying, "I do not want people to stare at me." What is the nurse's best response?

☐ 1. "That is OK for now if that's what you want."
☐ 2. "It will be easier for you if you face people as soon as possible."
☐ 3. "The staff are the only people who know why you were admitted."
☐ 4. "You are very hard on yourself."

CORRECT ANSWER: 4
The client is in the hospital for treatment, not for judgment. Option 1 avoids dealing with the client's feelings. Option 2 gives false reassurance. Option 3 is not necessarily true.

NP: Implementation
CN: Psychosocial integrity
CNS: Psychosocial adaptation
CL: Analysis

---

38 A 26-year-old office manager is hospitalized after developing acute leg pain. Diagnostic tests reveal no organic cause. What is the best long-term goal to include in this client's care planning?

☐ 1. Develop insight into the client's psyche.
☐ 2. Accelerate the client's developmental tasks.
☐ 3. Restore the client's previous adaptive behaviors.
☐ 4. Eliminate responsibility for the client's behavior.

CORRECT ANSWER: 3
The treatment team should identify ways to reduce the anxiety that caused the client's symptoms, develop more positive ways of managing the stress, and prevent secondary gains from the hospitalization. Conversion symptoms are not under voluntary control; they commonly represent a symbolic solution to an underlying conflict. Options 1, 2, and 4 are not closely related to the clinical picture of conversion disorder.

NP: Planning
CN: Psychosocial integrity
CNS: Coping and adaptation
CL: Analysis

39 A 16-year-old student has been admitted to your psychiatric unit after fainting in physical education class. She has a diagnosis of anorexia nervosa, weighs 88 lb (40 kg), and is 5′4″ (1.6 m) tall. She has been weighing herself several times a day at home and has lost 30 lb (13.5 kg) in the past 3 months. Which nursing diagnosis would be most appropriate for the client?

☐ 1. Altered thought processes
☐ 2. Impaired adjustment
☐ 3. Altered nutrition: less than body requirements
☐ 4. Altered sexuality patterns

CORRECT ANSWER: 3
Addressing the client's urgent physical needs is most important. Options 1, 2, and 4 are possible with anorexia nervosa, but no data in the case study directly support these diagnoses.
NP: Assessment
CN: Physiological integrity
CNS: Basic care and comfort
CL: Analysis

---

40 A client with antisocial personality disorder refuses to take a shower for 3 days. What is the nurse's best response?

☐ 1. "It is policy here for all clients to bathe daily."
☐ 2. "It is time for your shower. I will help you with it."
☐ 3. "Don't worry about your shower until tomorrow."
☐ 4. "Do you want people to make fun of you?"

CORRECT ANSWER: 2
This response offers support and sets limits. Option 1 does not offer support. Option 3 allows the client to continue to break rules. Option 4 offers neither support nor respect.
NP: Implementation
CN: Psychosocial integrity
CNS: Psychosocial adaptation
CL: Application

---

41 A client with major depression states, "Everything is my fault, and I would be better off dead." What is the priority nursing intervention?

☐ 1. Assess the seriousness of the client's comment.
☐ 2. Notify the psychiatrist of the client's verbalization.
☐ 3. Assign staff members to a suicide watch.
☐ 4. Engage the client in a no-suicide contract.

CORRECT ANSWER: 1
This situation demands an accurate assessment of the client's suicide potential. Options 2, 3, and 4 require more thorough assessment data before implementation.
NP: Assessment
CN: Psychosocial integrity
CNS: Psychosocial adaptation
CL: Analysis

42 An abused child is scheduled to be on the unit 3 to 4 weeks. Which of the following assignments would be best for the child?

☐ 1. Assign a different primary nurse to the child each day.
☐ 2. Assign the primary nurse who is transferring next week to another unit.
☐ 3. Assign the same primary nurse to the child each day of the hospital stay.
☐ 4. Assign a new primary nurse every 3 days.

CORRECT ANSWER: 3
This will provide continuity of care and allow trust to develop. Options 1, 2, and 4 are not in the best interest of the client and will not further a trusting relationship.
NP: Planning
CN: Safe, effective care environment
CNS: Management of care
CL: Application

---

43 A 38-year-old client is hospitalized with obsessive-compulsive disorder. On admission, she becomes nervous and asks to go to the bathroom to brush her teeth. Her husband says that she brushes her teeth at least 25 times a day. The nurse notes that the client's gums are inflamed and bleeding. Which is the best nursing intervention?

☐ 1. Have her stop brushing her teeth until the gums heal.
☐ 2. Allow her to continue her routine of daily brushing.
☐ 3. Monitor her dental care, and set limits on the amount of daily brushing.
☐ 4. Brush her teeth for her.

CORRECT ANSWER: 3
This allows the behavior that reduces anxiety for the client, but it sets limits as a first step in modifying the behavior. Option 1 may leave the client unable to manage anxiety. Option 2 does nothing to change the behavior. Option 4 treats the client like a toddler.
NP: Implementation
CN: Physiological integrity
CNS: Reduction of risk potential
CL: Application

---

44 A client with a diagnosis of organic mental disorder becomes verbally and physically abusive when the nurse enters the client's room to assist with daily care. Which of the following interventions should the nurse engage in first?

☐ 1. Check orders for physical and chemical restraints.
☐ 2. Set firm limits verbally.
☐ 3. Give clear directions while gently securing the client's arms from hitting the nurse.
☐ 4. Leave the room and let the angry, hostile behavior work itself out.

CORRECT ANSWER: 2
Clear limits protect the client, staff, and others. A verbally and physically abusive client sometimes responds to verbal controls. Option 1 may be carried out, but not as a first priority. The goal is to use the least restrictive intervention needed to reduce anxiety and control behavior. Restraints would be used only as a last resort. Option 3, an invasion of personal space, will likely escalate the hostile behavior. Additional staff help may be needed here. Option 4 could pose a safety problem. The client could fall or otherwise hurt herself in an attempt to strike out at the nurse or at an imagined threat.
NP: Implementation
CN: Safe, effective care environment
CNS: Safety and infection control
CL: Analysis

45 A $2^1/_2$-year-old client is hospitalized with a fractured left arm, a concussion, and multiple bruises. The client appears quite withdrawn. The bruises appear to have occurred at different times, with some new and some nearly healed. Emergency department staff report suspected child abuse to the authorities. During an assessment, the nurse would expect which behavior in the child?

☐ 1. Quiet and passive about pain
☐ 2. Crying and sensitive to pain
☐ 3. Happy to see new people
☐ 4. Having good eye contact with the parents

CORRECT ANSWER: 1
The abused child usually shows little emotion. Options 2, 3, and 4 describe conspicuous behavior that an abused child would typically avoid, for fear of provoking further abuse.
NP: Assessment
CN: Psychosocial integrity
CNS: Psychosocial adaptation
CL: Application

Mental Health Nursing

---

46 A bulimic client admitted to the psychiatric unit suddenly shouts, "I want to leave right now. I am not crazy and do not belong here." Which response should the nurse make?

☐ 1. "You cannot go home until we cure your eating problems."
☐ 2. "You seem upset; I will stay with you."
☐ 3. "Don't worry. You will feel better tomorrow."
☐ 4. "Let's talk about something more pleasant."

CORRECT ANSWER: 2
This response acknowledges the client's feelings and offers support. Option 1 fails to acknowledge the client's feelings, and the client probably cannot be kept against her will. Option 3 gives the client false reassurance and denies her feelings. Option 4 also denies the client's feelings.
NP: Implementation
CN: Psychosocial integrity
CNS: Psychosocial adaptation
CL: Application

---

47 A 22-year-old client has been diagnosed with antisocial personality disorder. She has been having problems since age 15, when she ran away from home. She has had two broken marriages, has been unable to keep a job for more than 2 months, and has had difficulties with the law because she has abused drugs and passed bad checks. Although the client has made all the telephone calls she is allowed for the day, she asks the nurse, "Can't I just make one more phone call?" What is the nurse's best response?

☐ 1. "Okay, but don't talk too long."
☐ 2. "Okay, if you promise to obey the rules the rest of the day."
☐ 3. "No, you can't. The rules apply equally to everyone, and you are asking to break them."
☐ 4. "No, you can't. Go watch television."

CORRECT ANSWER: 3
This response enforces the limits and explains why the client can't use the phone. Options 1 and 2 do not encourage the client to follow the rules. Option 4 does not explain why the client's request is being denied.
NP: Implementation
CN: Psychosocial integrity
CNS: Psychosocial adaptation
CL: Application

48 A client with anorexia nervosa who is on bed rest stares at her dinner tray. She has made little effort to eat. Which statement by the nurse would be most therapeutic?

☐ 1. "You should be ashamed of yourself. There are starving people who would love that food."
☐ 2. "Hurry up with your tray. I have several more clients to see."
☐ 3. "Don't worry. You can eat more tomorrow."
☐ 4. "I will stay with you while you eat and help you fill out tomorrow's menu."

CORRECT ANSWER: 4
This response shows that the nurse values the client, and it promotes eating by having the client select food preferences. Option 1 will not promote eating; in her weakened condition, the client probably does not care about world hunger. Option 2 implies that the nurse is too busy to spend time with the client. Option 3 placates the client and permits her to continue poor eating habits.
NP: Implementation
CN: Psychosocial integrity
CNS: Psychosocial adaptation
CL: Application

---

49 A client is hospitalized after experiencing sudden-onset paralysis. Diagnostic tests reveal no positive physical findings. What is a likely cause?

☐ 1. Demonstrated organic pathology
☐ 2. Intense feelings of worthlessness
☐ 3. A primary and conscious need for attention
☐ 4. An involuntary attempt to solve a conflict

CORRECT ANSWER: 4
In conversion disorder, the client unconsciously converts anxiety-provoking impulses into functional symptoms. Although primary gains occur (the anxiety-provoking impulse is avoided), the internal need or conflict is usually kept out of conscious awareness. Option 1: No physical pathology was discovered. Option 2: Anxiety, rather than feelings of worthlessness, is the primary motivator. Option 3: A hallmark of conversion disorder is that its attention-seeking activities are not conscious. The typical client cannot see the connection, obvious to others, between the anxiety-laden situation and the sudden illness that provides a means of escape.
NP: Assessment
CN: Psychosocial integrity
CNS: Coping and adaptation
CL: Comprehension

50 A 19-year-old male just arrived on the psychiatric unit from the emergency department. His medical diagnosis is personality disorder, and he exhibits manipulative behavior. As the nurse reviews the unit rules with him, the client asks, "Can I go to the snack shop just one time, and then I will answer whatever you want?" What is the nurse's best response?

- ☐ 1. "OK, but hurry up. I need to finish your assessment."
- ☐ 2. "OK, but only for 5 minutes."
- ☐ 3. "No, you can't go."
- ☐ 4. "No, you can't go. The rules here are for everyone."

CORRECT ANSWER: 4

This response sets limits with an appropriate explanation. Options 1 and 2 give in to the manipulative behavior. Option 3 does not explain the purpose of the refusal.

NP: Assessment
CN: Psychosocial integrity
CNS: Psychosocial adaptation
CL: Application

---

51 A client with major depression begins to improve and participates in treatment programs on the unit. The nurse should recognize that the client is ready for discharge when the client does which of the following?

- ☐ 1. Asks the staff for advice about how to handle the future
- ☐ 2. Speaks to the employer about a return date to work
- ☐ 3. Identifies personal weaknesses and plans to work on them
- ☐ 4. Discusses plans to return home and continue outpatient treatment

CORRECT ANSWER: 4

The client's plan to return home and continue treatment as an outpatient indicates responsibility for her own level of wellness. Asking the staff for advice (Option 1) implies that the client is still unable or unwilling to accept responsibility for herself. Although talking to her boss (Option 2) is a positive step, it will not help the client comprehensively. Identifying and working on weak areas (Option 3) represent short-term steps taken before discharge.

NP: Evaluation
CN: Psychosocial integrity
CNS: Coping and adaptation
CL: Analysis

52 Which of the following concepts about anorexia nervosa should the nurse consider in understanding a client's cry for help?

☐ 1. Focus on anorexia as an effort to gain status and resolve conflict
☐ 2. Rejection of food as a way to obtain love and care from parents
☐ 3. Use of eating behavior to resolve conscious sexual needs
☐ 4. Avoidance of eating as a response to voices that threaten the client

CORRECT ANSWER: 2
An anorexic client rigidly controls potentially disabling anxiety by controlling eating to the point of self-destructiveness. Conflicts most commonly encountered are issues of identity, separation, and autonomy; parents are commonly central figures in these struggles. Option 1: The function of anorexia nervosa as a means of dealing with anxiety is itself rooted in conflict. The client cannot seek resolution of the conflict without therapeutic intervention. Option 3: Far from embracing sexuality, the typical anorexic client stops menstruating, avoids adolescent sexual issues, and hides her body under baggy clothing. Option 4: An anorexic client usually does not experience hallucinations.

NP: Planning
CN: Psychosocial integrity
CNS: Psychosocial adaptation
CL: Analysis

---

53 A noticeably withdrawn 14-year-old female client is being treated on the unit for anorexia nervosa. Which nursing assessments should be made daily?

☐ 1. Edema of the legs
☐ 2. Pulse and blood pressure elevation
☐ 3. Frequent binging and purging
☐ 4. Level of depression and anxiety

CORRECT ANSWER: 4
Depression and anxiety commonly accompany anorexia nervosa. Options 1 and 2 are not associated with eating disorders. Option 3 is typical of bulimia.

NP: Assessment
CN: Psychosocial integrity
CNS: Psychosocial adaptation
CL: Application

---

54 A 76-year-old client is admitted to a long-term care facility with a diagnosis of organic mental disorder. The client has been wearing the same dirty, torn undergarments for several days. The nurse contacts family members to bring in clean clothing. Which of the following interventions would best prevent further regression in the client's personal hygiene habits?

☐ 1. Encourage the client to perform as much self-care as possible.
☐ 2. Make the client assume responsibility for physical care.
☐ 3. Assign a staff member to take over the client's physical care.
☐ 4. Accept the client's desire to go without bathing and to wear dirty clothing.

CORRECT ANSWER: 1
Clients with organically based problems tend to fluctuate in their capabilities. Encouraging self-care will help increase the client's orientation, provide a safe environment, and promote a trusting relationship with the nurse. Option 2 is unreasonable, given the client's possible confusion; self-esteem and independence must be developed as much as possible, but with assistance in activities of daily living. Option 3 restricts the client's independence. Option 4 would promote poor hygiene.

NP: Implementation
CN: Health promotion and maintenance
CNS: Prevention and early detection of disease
CL: Analysis

55 A 37-year-old man with a history of schizophrenia is having auditory hallucinations. He shouts to the nurse, "You are stepping on spiders! Move aside. Don't you see them?" What is the nurse's best response?

- ☐ 1. "No, I don't. Quit talking foolishly."
- ☐ 2. "Yes, I see them, and they sure are big ones."
- ☐ 3. "No, I don't see them, but I believe that you do see them."
- ☐ 4. "Let's go to the recreation room."

CORRECT ANSWER: 3

The nurse should present reality while acknowledging that the hallucination is real to the client. Option 1 presents reality but demeans the client in doing so. Option 2 encourages the client's hallucinations. Option 4 changes the subject and ignores the issue.

NP: Implementation
CN: Psychosocial integrity
CNS: Psychosocial adaptation
CL: Application

---

56 Teaching for a client taking antipsychotic medication should include which of the following instructions?

- ☐ 1. Take the medication with antacid to prevent upset stomach.
- ☐ 2. Get fresh air and plenty of sunshine.
- ☐ 3. If a dose is missed, take two the next time.
- ☐ 4. Avoid abrupt withdrawal of the medication.

CORRECT ANSWER: 4

Abrupt withdrawal could result in nausea or seizures. Option 1: Antacids decrease the effectiveness of antipsychotics when taken within 1 hour of the drug. Option 2: Because of the adverse effect of photosensitivity, clients taking antipsychotic drugs should avoid sun exposure. Option 3: Doubling up the medication could cause an overdose.

NP: Implementation
CN: Physiological integrity
CNS: Pharmacological and parenteral therapies
CL: Application

---

57 A client on an inpatient psychiatric unit at a community mental health center is pacing the hallway and appears agitated. When the nurse approaches him, he says loudly, "Leave me alone." What is the nurse's best approach?

- ☐ 1. Say "OK" and walk away.
- ☐ 2. Summon help in case the client becomes aggressive.
- ☐ 3. Say nothing and pace with the client.
- ☐ 4. Say, "You sound upset. I'd like to help."

CORRECT ANSWER: 4

This demonstrates the nurse's concern and encourages the client to discuss feelings. Option 1: Given the likelihood of an increase in anxiety level, the client should not be left alone. Option 2: Such an assumption of aggressiveness would probably escalate the client's anxiety. Option 3: This response does not acknowledge the client's emotional state.

NP: Implementation
CN: Psychosocial integrity
CNS: Psychosocial adaptation
CL: Analysis

58 A 23-year-old married homemaker has been on the psychiatric unit for 2 days. She has a history of bipolar disorder and came to the hospital in the manic phase. She stopped taking her medication (lithium carbonate [Eskalith]) 2 weeks ago. Which of the following findings would the nurse be least likely to see?

☐ 1. Flight of ideas
☐ 2. Delusions of grandeur
☐ 3. Increased appetite
☐ 4. Restlessness

CORRECT ANSWER: 3
The manic client is usually unwilling or unable to slow down enough to eat. Options 1, 2, and 4 are associated with the manic phase.
NP: Assessment
CN: Psychosocial integrity
CNS: Psychosocial adaptation
CL: Application

---

59 Which of the following instructions is most important for a client taking lithium carbonate [Eskalith]?

☐ 1. Limit fluids to 1½ qt (1,500 ml) daily.
☐ 2. Maintain a high fluid intake.
☐ 3. Take advantage of the warm weather by getting outside exercise when possible.
☐ 4. When feeling a cold coming on, take over-the-counter (OTC) medications.

CORRECT ANSWER: 2
Clients taking lithium need to maintain a high fluid intake. Option 1 is incorrect because fluids should not be limited. Option 3 is not safe; photosensitivity occurs with lithium use, and increased activity in warm weather could increase sodium loss, predisposing the client to a toxic reaction to lithium. Option 4 is incorrect because the client should not take OTC drugs without the physician's approval.
NP: Implementation
CN: Physiological integrity
CNS: Pharmacological and parenteral therapies
CL: Application

---

60 What is the best room assignment for a client with bipolar disorder, manic phase?

☐ 1. Alone, at the end of the hall
☐ 2. Alone, nearest the nurses' station
☐ 3. With another bipolar client at the end of the hall
☐ 4. With a depressed 40-year-old near the nurses' station

CORRECT ANSWER: 1
Such an assignment provides a quiet environment without the additional stimuli of a roommate and the noise of the nurses' station. Options 2, 3, and 4 provide too much stimulation and would likely increase the client's manic behavior.
NP: Planning
CN: Safe, effective care environment
CNS: Management of care
CL: Application

61 A 28-year-old single female arrives at a mental health clinic complaining of depression. She states that she has been feeling numb and empty most of the time and has little energy to perform her usual activities. She has experienced these difficulties since the death of her best friend 6 months ago. Which of the following is the nurse's best response?

☐ 1. Tell the client that the physician will prescribe an antidepressant and she will feel better.
☐ 2. Encourage the client to get on with her life and stop feeling sorry for herself.
☐ 3. Advise the client that it is not unusual for grieving and loss to continue for quite some time.
☐ 4. Suggest that the client return in 3 months if the feelings persist.

CORRECT ANSWER: 3
This provides the client with validation and support for her feelings. Options 1, 2, and 4 neither validate the client's bereavement nor allow her to resolve them.
NP: Implementation
CN: Psychosocial integrity
CNS: Coping and adaptation
CL: Application

---

62 A 50-year-old bookkeeper arrives for a follow-up visit after a severe wrist fracture 3 months ago. The tearful client expresses helplessness, frustration, and anxiety, stating that the injury was the worst experience of her life. The client's level of function is severely compromised. She has been unable to return to work and is currently receiving disability payments. What is the best response for the nurse to make?

☐ 1. "I can see how upsetting this is for you. It must be very difficult to be unable to function independently."
☐ 2. "I know how you must feel. I broke my arm a long time ago, but I am fine now. You will be as good as new soon."
☐ 3. "You are overly anxious. These injuries take time to heal, and you just have to be patient."
☐ 4. "I know it is difficult, but you'll just have to get hold of yourself and get on with your life."

CORRECT ANSWER: 1
This provides validation for the client's feelings. Options 2, 3, and 4 do not offer the client either support or the opportunity to discuss her feelings.
NP: Implementation
CN: Psychosocial integrity
CNS: Coping and adaptation
CL: Application

63 While making rounds in a senior citizens' housing complex, the visiting nurse discovers one of her clients sobbing in her darkened apartment. On questioning the client, an 85-year-old widow, the nurse learns that her pet cat of 15 years had been put to sleep the day before. Which is the best response for the nurse to make?

- ☐ 1. "It shouldn't be hard to find another cat. You will feel better once you have another pet."
- ☐ 2. "It was only a cat. Why are you allowing yourself to be so upset? It would be different if it were a person."
- ☐ 3. "I'm so sorry that your pet had to be put to sleep. I know how important your cat was to you."
- ☐ 4. "It's probably best for the cat because it was so old and ill."

CORRECT ANSWER: 3

This offers support and empathy and enhances the grieving process. Options 1, 2, and 4 do not address the client's need for support and grieving.

NP: Implementation
CN: Psychosocial integrity
CNS: Coping and adaptation
CL: Application

---

64 A 42-year-old homemaker presents in the emergency department with uncontrollable tension and anxiety, difficulty in eating and sleeping, and feelings of extreme insecurity. Her husband of 17 years has recently asked for a divorce. The client is crying hysterically and rocking in a chair. Which is the best response for the nurse to make?

- ☐ 1. "You must stop crying so that we can discuss your feelings about the divorce."
- ☐ 2. "Once you find a job, you will feel much better and more secure."
- ☐ 3. "I can see how upset you are. Let's sit in the office so that we can talk about how you are feeling."
- ☐ 4. "Once you have a lawyer looking out for your interests, you will feel better."

CORRECT ANSWER: 3

This response validates the client's distress and provides an opportunity to talk about her feelings. Because clients in crisis have difficulty making decisions, the nurse must be directive as well as supportive. Option 1 does not provide the client with adequate support. Options 2 and 4 do not acknowledge the client's distress. Moreover, clients in crisis cannot think beyond the immediate moment, so discussing long-range plans is not helpful.

NP: Implementation
CN: Psychosocial integrity
CNS: Psychosocial adaptation
CL: Application

65 A 35-year-old married truck driver presents at a mental health clinic. Since losing his job 2 weeks ago, he has slept only a few hours a night and has lost 10 lb (4.5 kg). Pale and haggard, he has trouble answering questions and is easily distracted. Which is the best action for the nurse to take?

☐ 1. Ask him if he has tried to find another job.
☐ 2. Determine his current and previous level of function and conduct a mental status examination.
☐ 3. Ask him if he has ever sought mental health counseling before and whether or not he is taking any medications.
☐ 4. Ask about his family's reaction to his job loss.

CORRECT ANSWER: 2

This action assesses the client's current level of function, emotional state, and stability. Options 1, 3, and 4 do not offer the client support or assist in evaluating his current status.

NP: Assessment
CN: Psychosocial integrity
CNS: Psychosocial adaptation
CL: Application

---

66 A 50-year-old single male is brought to the crisis unit by the police after having escaped unharmed from his apartment, which was destroyed by a fire caused by his smoking in bed. The nurse observes the client sitting silently, almost motionless. Several other clients in the waiting room have commented about the heavy odor of smoke around the man. Which of the following is the nurse's best approach to the client?

☐ 1. "Would you like to change your clothes? The odor of smoke must be very disturbing."
☐ 2. "You have been through a very difficult experience. Let's move into the office so that we can talk."
☐ 3. "I hope you have learned your lesson today and have given up cigarettes."
☐ 4. "You must consider yourself one very lucky man."

CORRECT ANSWER: 2

The client is immobilized by his near-death experience, the loss of his home, and his responsibility for these situations based on his smoking. Because he cannot make decisions at this point, the nurse's direction is appropriate and therapeutic. It also provides a tactful way to alleviate the odor of smoke in the waiting room. Options 1, 3, and 4 do not provide support or direction for the client during this crisis.

NP: Assessment
CN: Psychosocial integrity
CNS: Coping and adaptation
CL: Application

67 A 19-year-old nursing student preparing for final exams arrives at the student health center, accompanied by two friends. She has not slept all night, is sobbing hysterically, is hyperventilating, and states that she "cannot go on." Which of the following is the best response for the nurse to make?

- ☐ 1. "Relax, we've all felt this way. You'll get through it."
- ☐ 2. "Perhaps you need more time to study. Have you discussed this with your advisor?"
- ☐ 3. "You're pretty upset right now. Studying for finals can be very stressful. Let's work on a plan that might be helpful."
- ☐ 4. "You need to calm down. Nurses have to learn to take a lot of stress."

CORRECT ANSWER: 3

This provides support, reassurance, and a concrete plan for dealing with the issues. Option 1 provides false reassurance. Option 2 is unrealistic; a client in high anxiety cannot think coherently enough to respond to such a suggestion. Option 4 negates the client's feelings and may cause further anxiety.

NP: Implementation
CN: Psychosocial integrity
CNS: Coping and adaptation
CL: Application

---

68 A 26-year-old single woman is knocked down and robbed while walking her dog one evening. Three months later, she presents at the crisis clinic, stating that she cannot put this experience out of her mind. She complains of nightmares, extreme fear of being outside or alone, and difficulty eating and sleeping. What is the best response for the nurse to make?

- ☐ 1. "I will ask the physician to prescribe medication for you."
- ☐ 2. "That must have been a very difficult and frightening experience. It might be helpful to talk about it."
- ☐ 3. "In the future, you might walk your dog in a more populated area or hire someone else to take over this task."
- ☐ 4. "Have you thought of moving to a safer neighborhood?"

CORRECT ANSWER: 2

The client receives support and an opportunity to discuss the experience. Options 1, 3, and 4 do not validate her experience or permit discussion of feelings.

NP: Implementation
CN: Psychosocial integrity
CNS: Coping and adaptation
CL: Application

69 A 60-year-old widower is hospitalized after complaining of difficulty sleeping, extreme apprehension, shortness of breath, and a sense of impending doom. What is the best response for the nurse to make?

- ☐ 1. "You have nothing to worry about. You are in a safe place. Try to relax."
- ☐ 2. "Has anything happened recently or in the past that may have triggered these feelings?"
- ☐ 3. "We have given you a medication that will help to decrease these feelings of anxiety."
- ☐ 4. "Take some deep breaths and try and calm down."

CORRECT ANSWER: 2

This provides support, reassurance, and an opportunity to gain insight into the cause of the anxiety. Option 1 dismisses the client's feelings and offers false reassurance. Options 3 and 4 do not allow the client to discuss his feelings, which he must do in order to understand and resolve the cause of his anxiety.

NP: Implementation
CN: Psychosocial integrity
CNS: Psychosocial adaptation
CL: Application

---

70 A 45-year-old lawyer has been hospitalized because of severe agitation. He feels that he must pace the floor a specific number of times each day or something "terrible" will happen to him. He has engaged in this behavior most of his adult life. What is the most therapeutic response for the nurse to make?

- ☐ 1. "Nothing will happen to you. You must stop this behavior."
- ☐ 2. "Are you looking for attention? There are other ways you can get it."
- ☐ 3. "This behavior has created some difficulty for you. It might help if we talked about why you find it necessary to do this."
- ☐ 4. ""I will have the physician prescribe medication that will help you stop pacing."

CORRECT ANSWER: 3

This provides a structure for reducing the client's anxiety, gaining insight into his behavior, and eventually redirecting the anxiety. Options 1, 2, and 4 do not assist the client in gaining insight and may actually increase his anxiety.

NP: Implementation
CN: Psychosocial integrity
CNS: Psychosocial adaptation
CL: Application

71 A 59-year-old married woman comes to the mental health clinic after experiencing panic attacks. She has been unable to drive her car or leave her home alone since she lost her job several weeks ago. She complains of palpitations, sweating, shortness of breath, and fear of impending doom. What would be the nurse's best response?

- ☐ 1. "You must try to leave your home each day for a brief period of time."
- ☐ 2. "These symptoms will decrease if you work on them, avoid drinking coffee, and stop smoking."
- ☐ 3. "You are experiencing panic attacks. Perhaps we can help you to understand why these attacks are occurring."
- ☐ 4. "You need to calm down so that you will be able to find another job."

CORRECT ANSWER: 3

This assists the client in gaining insight into the cause or origin of the attacks, a necessary first step in resolving them. Options 1 and 4 do not validate the client's experience. Option 2 offers concrete strategies that cannot be applied effectively until the client gains insight into the cause of the attacks.

NP: Implementation
CN: Psychosocial integrity
CNS: Psychosocial adaptation
CL: Application

---

72 A 26-year-old male is admitted to an inpatient psychiatric hospital after having been picked up by the local police while walking around the neighborhood at night without shoes in the snow. He appears confused and disoriented. Which of the following is the most immediate nursing action?

- ☐ 1. Assess and stabilize the client's medical needs.
- ☐ 2. Assess and stabilize the client's psychiatric needs.
- ☐ 3. Attempt to locate the nearest family members to get an accurate history.
- ☐ 4. Arrange a transfer to the nearest medical facility.

CORRECT ANSWER: 1

The possibility of frostbite must be evaluated before the other interventions. Options 2, 3, and 4 do not address the client's immediate medical needs.

NP: Implementation
CN: Physiological integrity
CNS: Physiological adaptation
CL: Analysis

---

73 A client with decreased mental capacity from dementia is being admitted to a nursing home. Which of the following actions should take priority for the nurse?

- ☐ 1. Provide a safe environment free from hazards.
- ☐ 2. Provide the family with information about nursing home placement and costs.
- ☐ 3. Orient family members to the nursing home, and show them where they can put their things.
- ☐ 4. Administer the prescribed medications.

CORRECT ANSWER: 1

A safe environment is essential when a client has decreased mental capacity. Options 2 and 3 provide important information for the family, but they do not address the client's decreased mental capacity. Option 4 is incorrect because no medication is currently available to treat dementia, and some medications can worsen it.

NP: Implementation
CN: Safe, effective care environment
CNS: Safety and infection control
CL: Application

74 Which of the following actions is most important to include in the treatment plan for a schizophrenic client?

☐ 1. Posting a daily schedule for the client to follow
☐ 2. Attending education classes on hygiene and illness
☐ 3. Establishing goals and objectives
☐ 4. Promoting individual therapy

CORRECT ANSWER: 3

Goals and objectives are the basis of treatment for any client. Options 1, 2, and 3 may all be incorporated into goals and objectives.

NP: Planning
CN: Psychosocial integrity
CNS: Psychosocial adaptation
CL: Application

---

75 A 45-year-old housewife has been treated for major depression for the past 15 years. Her physician has recently prescribed an MAO inhibitor. Which of the following foods should the nurse instruct the client to avoid?

☐ 1. Smoked salmon
☐ 2. Milk and eggs
☐ 3. Honey
☐ 4. Dried nuts

CORRECT ANSWER: 1

Smoked foods contain tyramine, a substance that can produce a hypertensive crisis in a client taking an MAO inhibitor. Options 2, 3, and 4 do not contain tyramine.

NP: Planning
CN: Physiological integrity
CNS: Pharmacological and parenteral therapies
CL: Application

---

76 A client taking an MAO inhibitor should receive instructions about the adverse reaction associated with tyramine. Which of the following drug-drug interactions should the nurse discuss with the client?

☐ 1. Aspirin
☐ 2. Anticoagulants
☐ 3. Antihistamines
☐ 4. Antihypertensives

CORRECT ANSWER: 4

One of the adverse effects of MAO inhibitors is hypotension. If this occurs in a client already taking antihypertensive medication, heart failure can result. Options 1, 2, and 3 do not produce a drug-drug interaction with MAO inhibitors.

NP: Planning
CN: Physiological integrity
CNS: Pharmacological and parenteral therapies
CL: Application

---

77 A 70-year-old widow has been diagnosed with Alzheimer's disease. She has lived alone with little difficulty since her husband died 5 years ago. Recently, however, her daughter has observed the client's inability to comprehend or express herself verbally, echolalia, and a tendency to wander the neighborhood. Based on the nurse's confirmation of these signs, which stage of the disease is the client experiencing?

☐ 1. Stage I
☐ 2. Stage II
☐ 3. Stage III
☐ 4. Stage IV

CORRECT ANSWER: 2

The listed behaviors are associated with stage II, an advancing stage of Alzheimer's disease. Behaviors associated with stage I focus on emotional and memory problems. Stage III is characterized by an additional inability to maintain physiologic functions. There is no stage IV.

NP: Assessment
CN: Psychosocial integrity
CNS: Psychosocial adaptation
CL: Application

78 A client on an MAO inhibitor demonstrates that learning has taken place by naming tyramine-containing foods and by relating that even moderate amounts of tyramine must be avoided to prevent a hypertensive crisis. The client would be correct in naming which of the following foods?

- ☐ 1. Swiss cheese
- ☐ 2. Cream cheese
- ☐ 3. Milk
- ☐ 4. Ice cream

CORRECT ANSWER: 1

Fermented, aged, pickled, or smoked foods tend to be high in tyramine. Options 2, 3, and 4 are unfermented milk products that may be taken without problems.

NP: Evaluation
CN: Physiological integrity
CNS: Pharmacological and parenteral therapies
CL: Application

---

79 A woman is trying to cope after the sudden death of her husband during emergency heart surgery. Which of the following statements by the wife would indicate the isolation stage of grieving?

- ☐ 1. "Why can't you people do something to keep him alive?"
- ☐ 2. "What is the use of going on without him?"
- ☐ 3. "If only I could have seen him one more time and told him that I loved him."
- ☐ 4. "Oh, no! He can't be dead!"

CORRECT ANSWER: 4

This answer indicates shock and disbelief, common with the denial and isolation stage of grieving. The blame and frustration expressed in Option 1 indicate the anger stage. The hopelessness evident in Option 2 indicates the depression stage. "If only . . ." statements (Option 3) typify the bargaining stage.

NP: Assessment
CN: Psychosocial integrity
CNS: Coping and adaptation
CL: Analysis

---

80 A 25-year-old male with a history of bipolar disorder is admitted to the acute care psychiatric unit of a local hospital after having spent the family's savings on a luxury automobile. The client had been taking 300 mg of lithium carbonate (Eskalith) three times a day, but he stopped 4 weeks before his hospitalization. Which of the following would take priority in the client's plan of care?

- ☐ 1. Serum lithium levels should be drawn weekly throughout treatment.
- ☐ 2. The client should maintain a balanced diet and salt intake.
- ☐ 3. The client should avoid driving a car because of lithium's sedative effects.
- ☐ 4. The client's physician should prescribe the sustained-release version of lithium to enhance compliance.

CORRECT ANSWER: 2

A delicate balance between sodium intake and lithium must be maintained to avoid a toxic reaction. Option 1: Serum lithium levels need to be drawn weekly only until maintenance levels have been reached. Option 3: The sedative action of lithium is only an initial adverse effect. Option 4: The sustained-release form of lithium would not be an initial concern of the nurse.

NP: Planning
CN: Physiological integrity
CNS: Pharmacological and parenteral therapies
CL: Application

81 Lithium carbonate (Eskalith) takes 1 to 2 weeks to reach its therapeutic level. Which of the following drugs would a nurse expect the physician to prescribe to help control a client's manic behavior?

☐ 1. Haloperidol (Haldol)
☐ 2. Imipramine (Tofranil)
☐ 3. Chlorpromazine (Thorazine)
☐ 4. Diazepam (Valium)

CORRECT ANSWER: 3
Chlorpromazine, an antipsychotic medication, will help control the client's behavior. Although haloperidol (Option 1) is an antipsychotic, its use with lithium holds the possibility of a drug-drug interaction. Imipramine (Option 2) is an antidepressant. Diazepam (Option 4) is an antianxiety drug.

NP: Planning
CN: Physiological integrity
CNS: Pharmacological and parenteral therapies
CL: Analysis

---

82 A nurse is teaching a client and family about compliance with lithium carbonate (Eskalith) therapy. Which of the following actions should the nurse recommend if the client is required to take the drug three times a day and she misses a single dose?

☐ 1. Take two doses of lithium at the next scheduled time.
☐ 2. Skip the remaining doses for the day.
☐ 3. Take the remaining doses as prescribed.
☐ 4. Take all the prescribed doses at once.

CORRECT ANSWER: 3
This allows for medication compliance without a high risk of toxic reaction because lithium's half-life is 24 hours. Doubling or tripling the prescribed dosage (Options 1 and 4) would place the client at extreme risk for a toxic reaction. Skipping doses (Option 2) may reduce therapeutic drug levels.

NP: Implementation
CN: Physiological integrity
CNS: Pharmacological and parenteral therapies
CL: Application

---

83 A 33-year-old male is admitted to the hospital for depression. He is actively suicidal. The physician has prescribed phenelzine (Nardil). After the nurse reviews dietary restrictions, what would be the next most important information to give the client?

☐ 1. "It may take as long as 3 weeks for the drug to take effect."
☐ 2. "If you notice any unpleasant side effects like dizziness, report it immediately to the nurse."
☐ 3. "Once you start taking the medication, you will begin to feel better."
☐ 4. "You will still need to be on suicide precautions for your own safety."

CORRECT ANSWER: 1
Phenelzine can take up to 3 weeks before its therapeutic effects work for depression. MAO must be inhibited at receptor sites to permit an increase in neurotransmitters such as epinephrine, norepinephrine, and dopamine. Giving the client information about adverse effects that are not life-threatening (Option 2) is not as important as telling him how long he may have to wait for the drug to take effect against depression. Option 3 gives false reassurance; the effects may not be felt for 3 weeks and, in any case, cannot be guaranteed. Option 4 does not relate to the teaching plan for phenelzine.

NP: Implementation
CN: Physiological integrity
CNS: Pharmacological and parenteral therapies
CL: Analysis

84 A 24-year-old female catatonic schizophrenic is admitted to the unit in a catatonic state. She is placed on 5 mg of haloperidol (Haldol) three times a day. Four days after her admission, she comes out of her coma and slowly begins to take care of herself. She says that the F.B.I. is after her because she was a key figure in the Iran-contra affair with Oliver North. What is the nurse's best response?

☐ 1. "How long have you known Oliver North?"
☐ 2. "You do not know Oliver North."
☐ 3. "Why do you think the F.B.I. would be looking for you here?"
☐ 4. "You must feel important. Can I accompany you to breakfast?"

CORRECT ANSWER: 4
This answer first addresses the underlying need for which the delusion may be created and then redirects the client's focus to a current, reality-based situation. Asking about the delusion (Options 1 and 3) reinforces it and does not help the client give it up. Option 2 directly challenges the delusion, which will probably prompt the client to cling to it more tightly.
NP: Implementation
CN: Psychosocial integrity
CNS: Psychosocial adaptation
CL: Analysis

---

85 Observing a delusional client talking to herself on the unit, the nurse determines that she is hallucinating. What is the most important information to gather next?

☐ 1. Vital signs
☐ 2. Whether the voices are telling her to harm herself
☐ 3. Whether she is talking to someone she sees on the unit
☐ 4. Level of antipsychotic medication in her bloodstream

CORRECT ANSWER: 2
The most important action is to assess the safety of a client who is actively hallucinating. If the voices are telling her to harm herself, the nurse needs to know. Vital signs (Option 1) are not significantly altered in a harmful way during a hallucination. Option 3 does not deal with safety issues and is therefore not a priority to assess. The client's medication (Option 4) may or may not need adjustment, but safety must be the immediate priority.
NP: Assessment
CN: Safe, effective care environment
CNS: Safety and infection control
CL: Analysis

86 A 66-year-old woman, diagnosed with dementia, is placed in a nursing home because caring for her at home has become difficult for the family. She had been wandering off from the house and was found in the middle of the highway, wearing only her nightgown. Which of the following measures should be included in her nursing care?

☐ 1. Assessing her vital signs
☐ 2. Assessing the family's guilt at placing her in a nursing home
☐ 3. Restraining the client according to hospital policy
☐ 4. Providing constant supervision

Correct answer: 4

Because of the severity of her dementia, the client requires constant supervision. She should not be left alone even for short periods. Option 1 is important client information, but it is not as important as ensuring the client's safety. Although guilt (Option 2) is a common reaction for families who must place a loved one in a nursing home, the information given here does not suggest that this family feels guilty. Option 3 is a common practice in clinical settings, all too often for the nurse's convenience rather than the client's safety.

NP: Planning
CN: Psychosocial integrity
CNS: Psychosocial adaptation
CL: Application

---

87 A nurse is performing a mental health assessment on a confused and disoriented client. Which of the following would best help the nurse assess the client's abstract thinking skills?

☐ 1. Ask the client to explain the proverb "A rolling stone gathers no moss."
☐ 2. Ask the client to respond to a hypothetical situation, such as, "What would you do if you found a letter with the stamp affixed?"
☐ 3. Ask the client to name the last five presidents of the United States.
☐ 4. Ask the client to identify the reason for being admitted to the hospital.

Correct answer: 1

This requires the client to draw conclusions based on commonly available information. Option 2 is best used to test for reasoning and judgment. Option 3 tests for knowledge of a general fund of information. Option 4 tests for insight.

NP: Assessment
CN: Psychosocial integrity
CNS: Psychosocial adaptation
CL: Application

---

88 A 25-year-old male schizophrenic has just been transferred to the unit from the forensic hospital. The client states, "I was in prison because I attempted to kill a policeman." What is the nurse's best therapeutic response?

☐ 1. "Why did you do that?"
☐ 2. "Did he try to hurt you?"
☐ 3. "Kill a policeman."
☐ 4. "What medication are you taking?"

Correct answer: 3

Restating shows that the client's words were heard and understood. "Why" questions (Option 1) can make clients angry. Option 2 is a closed, leading question. Option 4 changes the focus.

NP: Assessment
CN: Psychosocial integrity
CNS: Psychosocial adaptation
CL: Application

Mental Health Nursing

89 A 45-year-old man is brought into the emergency department after suffering a heart attack and losing control of his truck. Despite the efforts of emergency personnel at the scene and hospital staff members, the client dies. A physician has just informed the client's wife. What is the nurse's best response while comforting the wife?

☐ 1. "The physician and emergency team did all that they could to save your husband."
☐ 2. "Can I go with you to the chapel and sit with you for a while?"
☐ 3. "Let me call your chaplain to help you."
☐ 4. "I wouldn't recommend you see him until the funeral home has had time to prepare the body."

CORRECT ANSWER: 2
This response offers the nurse's support in a quiet environment and allows time for the wife to adjust to her husband's sudden death. Option 1 may help the nurse feel better, but it does not show awareness of what the wife is experiencing. Option 3 presumes, perhaps incorrectly, that the wife has a chaplain and that she would find comfort in his presence. Option 4 fails to recognize that seeing her husband's body would allow the wife to begin the necessary grieving process.

NP: Implementation
CN: Psychosocial integrity
CNS: Coping and adaptation
CL: Analysis

---

90 Which cognitive change would the nurse expect to find after completing a mental health assessment on a client with Alzheimer's disease?

☐ 1. Loss of recent memory
☐ 2. Total memory loss
☐ 3. Loss of remote memory
☐ 4. No memory loss

CORRECT ANSWER: 1
Recent memory loss supports the presence of an organic disorder. Options 2, 3, and 4 usually do not.

NP: Assessment
CN: Psychosocial integrity
CNS: Psychosocial adaptation
CL: Application

---

91 About 18 months after his wife's sudden death, the husband is speaking to a nurse about his current feelings. Which of the following statements by the husband would indicate that he had resolved the grieving process?

☐ 1. "I wish I could have seen her one more time."
☐ 2. "I think it's time for me to rejoin my bridge club."
☐ 3. "I could not possibly marry anyone else but her."
☐ 4. "I still occasionally set the table with two plates, but I'm getting better about setting the table for just one."

CORRECT ANSWER: 2
The husband is showing a readiness to rejoin the social world. After a loss, isolation is common as the bereaved one goes through the stages of grieving. Rejoining the social world suggests that acceptance has occurred. Option 1 indicates that the husband is still in the bargaining phase of grieving. Option 3 suggests that the husband is not progressing through the various stages. He also may feel extreme loyalty to his wife and extreme guilt that he was unable to say goodbye. Option 4 suggests that the husband is recovering but that he may still be in the depression stage of grieving.

NP: Evaluation
CN: Psychosocial integrity
CNS: Coping and adaptation
CL: Analysis

92 A 75-year-old widow is perceived by her family as "doing well" at the funeral of her husband, who lived with a diagnosis of terminal cancer for 2 years while undergoing various experimental treatments. Family members ask the home health nurse for an explanation of their mother's reaction at their father's funeral. What is the nurse's best response?

- ☐ 1. "He is in a better place, and she knows this."
- ☐ 2. "Your mother is denying the reality of her husband's death and needs your support."
- ☐ 3. "Your mother is not acting appropriately for someone of her age who is grieving; she needs a mental health center referral."
- ☐ 4. "Your mother had some time for anticipatory grieving over the past 2 years and was sort of prepared for his death."

Correct answer: 4

The husband's long illness and various treatments allowed the widow to prepare somewhat for his death and to engage in anticipatory grieving. Option 1 gives the family false reassurance. Strong denial (Option 2) is more likely when the death is sudden. No information in this case study suggests that the widow's grieving is abnormal or that she needs a mental health referral (Option 3).

NP: Implementation
CN: Psychosocial integrity
CNS: Coping and adaptation
CL: Analysis

---

93 A 33-year-old male nurse is admitted to the hospital unit with a diagnosis of delirium. In preparing to provide nursing care to him, the nurse should assess which of the following factors first?

- ☐ 1. The interplay of emotions and physical reactions
- ☐ 2. The pathophysiological processes leading to brain hypoxia
- ☐ 3. The psychopathological changes leading to confusion
- ☐ 4. The intrapsychic changes resulting from dysfunctional family interactions

Correct answer: 2

Hypoxia causes changes in brain physiology, which can lead to delirium. Option 1: Although emotions produce a response in the physical realm, the response does not lead to delirium. Option 3: Psychopathology refers to psychological changes; delirium has a physiological basis. Option 4: Negative family dynamics are not a factor in producing delirium.

NP: Assessment
CN: Physiological integrity
CNS: Physiological adaptation
CL: Application

---

94 Which of the following principles takes priority when planning the use of restraints on nursing home residents?

- ☐ 1. The use of restraints decreases the incidence of falls in nursing homes.
- ☐ 2. The use of restraints does not decrease the incidence of falls in nursing homes.
- ☐ 3. No serious injuries resulting from the use of restraints have been documented.
- ☐ 4. Elderly clients tend to feel more secure when a restraint is in place.

Correct answer: 2

The use of restraints in nursing homes increases the incidence of falls and serious injuries (such as abrasions, vasoconstriction, nerve damage, chest constriction, and breathing problems). In most instances, restraints do not make a client feel more secure, but rather bring about more confusion, frustration, and despair, sometimes even robbing the client of the will to live.

NP: Planning
CN: Safe, effective care environment
CNS: Safety and infection control
CL: Application

95 A 43-year-old paranoid schizophrenic is hospitalized in the psychiatric unit. Lately, he has thought that microwaves were broadcasting to his television set about hostile forces poised to invade, and he has placed aluminum foil over his windows and around his ankles so that they cannot track him after the invasion. He observes two nursing students talking and asks his nurse why they are talking about him. What is the nurse's best response?

☐ 1. "The students are studying to be good nurses. You should not be afraid of them."

☐ 2. "The students will stop talking to each other if you like."

☐ 3. "Why do you think the students are talking about you?"

☐ 4. "You sound frightened. I'll sit with you while you have breakfast."

CORRECT ANSWER: 4

This response avoids reinforcing the client's idea of reference, acknowledges the client's fearful feelings, and redirects him to the here and now. Option 1 is defensive and gives the client advice. Option 2 reinforces the client's idea of reference. Option 3 is a "why" question that the client may perceive as overly demanding or even threatening.

NP: Implementation
CN: Psychosocial integrity
CNS: Psychosocial adaptation
CL: Analysis

Maternal-Infant Nursing

1 A client with hypotonic labor dysfunction has been started on oxytocin (Pitocin). Despite adequate contractions, the fetus does not descend lower than 0 station. The physician recommends cesarean delivery. The client and her husband are confused because she had given birth previously to an average-size infant. They ask several questions about cesarean birth. What would be the most accurate nursing diagnosis for this client?

- ☐ 1. Anger related to loss of planned birth experience
- ☐ 2. Anxiety related to lack of knowledge about the need for cesarean birth
- ☐ 3. Pain related to long, unproductive labor
- ☐ 4. Fear related to the unknown

Correct answer: 2

The couple's questions indicate their lack of knowledge. Anxiety is expected because a cesarean delivery was unplanned. Options 1, 3, and 4 are not indicated by the stated assessment data.

NP: Assessment
CN: Health promotion and maintenance
CNS: Prevention and early detection of disease
CL: Analysis

---

2 What is the best way to teach new parents about the care of their infant?

- ☐ 1. Relate stories of other parents' experiences.
- ☐ 2. Focus on the behavior of their own infant.
- ☐ 3. Show videotapes about newborn care.
- ☐ 4. Distribute literature with photographs of infant-care skills.

Correct answer: 2

Working directly with the parents' newborn offers the best opportunity for the nurse to demonstrate infant-care techniques and elicit return demonstration by the parents. Pointing out specific behaviors and characteristics of their baby enhances parent-infant attachment. Options 1, 3, and 4 are less meaningful teaching methods.

NP: Planning
CN: Health promotion and maintenance
CNS: Growth and development through the life span
CL: Application

3 A girl, delivered at 38 weeks' gestation, weighs 5 lb, 2 oz. She is having difficulty maintaining body temperature. Her mother had pregnancy-induced hypertension (PIH). The baby develops acrocyanosis of the extremities on the evening of her birth. The nurse should know that this is not a dangerous sign for which of the following reasons?

☐ 1. This condition may be related to the baby's temperature instability.
☐ 2. Blue extremities may reflect a lower level of hemoglobin present in babies of mothers with PIH.
☐ 3. Vasomotor instability causes venous blood to move readily through the circulatory system, resulting in acrocyanosis.
☐ 4. Acrocyanosis is usual for newborns and may last up to 6 months.

CORRECT ANSWER: 1
Cold stress commonly increases acrocyanosis in newborns. Option 2: Newborns usually have a high level of hemoglobin, which is not affected by PIH. Option 3: Venous stasis decreases blood flow from the extremities. Option 4: Acrocyanosis in the newborn is transient.

NP: Assessment
CN: Physiological integrity
CNS: Reduction of risk potential
CL: Analysis

---

4 A 26-year-old Type 1 diabetic in the second trimester of pregnancy has been hospitalized for diabetes management. She performs blood glucose testing at 6 a.m., 11 a.m., 4 p.m., and 9 p.m. At 8 a.m. the client receives NPH and regular insulins subcutaneously. A dextrose paste is kept at bedside, and the client has been instructed to report symptoms of hypoglycemia. At 4 p.m. the client obtains a blood glucose reading of 45 mg/dl. As instructed, she notifies the nurse. What is the nurse's first response?

☐ 1. Administer insulin.
☐ 2. Notify the physician.
☐ 3. Provide the client with a glass of skim milk.
☐ 4. No nursing action is warranted at this time.

CORRECT ANSWER: 3
A blood glucose level of 45 mg/dl indicates hypoglycemia. Skim milk will increase the blood glucose level. Administering additional insulin (Option 1) would further decrease the blood glucose level. Notifying the physician (Option 2) would be appropriate only after treating the hypoglycemia. Performing no nursing action (Option 4) may harm the client and her fetus.

NP: Implementation
CN: Physiological integrity
CNS: Reduction of risk potential
CL: Analysis

5 A woman in her 8th month of pregnancy is having dinner with her husband at their favorite restaurant. The woman suddenly chokes on a piece of chicken and appears to lose consciousness. What would be the best action by a nurse sitting at the next table?

☐ 1. Apply abdominal thrust.
☐ 2. Apply chest thrust.
☐ 3. Begin cardiopulmonary resuscitation.
☐ 4. Reposition the client on her side.

CORRECT ANSWER: 2

Because it prevents fetal injury, a chest thrust is the best way to force air through the throat and dislodge the obstruction. Option 1 might cause fetal injury. Options 3 and 4 would not help dislodge the obstruction.

NP: Implementation
CN: Physiological integrity
CNS: Physiological adaptation
CL: Application

---

6 A client in labor has received an epidural of bupivacaine hydrochloride (Sensorcaine) and epinephrine. Which of the following conditions would take highest priority in a nursing assessment?

☐ 1. Hypertension
☐ 2. Hypotension
☐ 3. Polyuria
☐ 4. Oliguria

CORRECT ANSWER: 2

An epidural block acts similarly to spinal anesthesia. Both can produce hypotension by blocking the sympathetic division of the autonomic nervous system. Hypertension (Option 1) does not result from an epidural block. Polyuria (Option 3) is not an effect of an epidural block. Oliguria (Option 4) could occur as a result of hypotension, but it would not be the client's first response.

NP: Assessment
CN: Physiological integrity
CNS: Pharmacological and parenteral therapies
CL: Analysis

---

7 A Type 1 diabetic in the second trimester of pregnancy is consuming a 2,400-calorie American Diabetes Association diet divided into three meals and several snacks. Her breakfast meal plan consists of these exchanges: 3 breads, 1 meat, 1 fruit, 1 milk, and 2 fats. Which of the following menus would best comply with the meal plan?

☐ 1. One English muffin, 1/2 cup cooked grits, 1 egg, 1/2 banana, 1 cup skim milk, and 2 tsp margarine
☐ 2. Two bagels (1/2 bagel per exchange), 1 cup cooked grits, 3 eggs, 1 banana, 1 cup whole milk, 3 tsp margarine
☐ 3. Four breadsticks, 1 oz ham, 1 small apple, 2 slices bacon, and 1 cup low-fat yogurt
☐ 4. Three breadsticks, 2 oz ham, 30 grapes (15 grapes per exchange), and 2 tsp fat

CORRECT ANSWER: 1

This menu includes the following exchanges: 3 breads (two halves of the English muffin plus 1/2 cup cooked grits), 1 meat (1 egg), 1 fruit (1/2 banana), 1 milk (1 cup skim milk), and 2 fats (2 tsp margarine). Option 2 exceeds the bread, meat, and fat exchanges. Option 3 exceeds the bread exchanges. Option 4 exceeds the meat and fruit exchanges.

NP: Implementation
CN: Physiological integrity
CNS: Basic care and comfort
CL: Analysis

8 A primigravida client with acquired immunodeficiency syndrome (AIDS) is in labor at term. In preparing her nursing care plan, the nurse should include which of the following nursing diagnoses?

☐ 1. Risk for fetal or maternal injury related to the crisis of childbearing
☐ 2. Risk for infection related to suppressed immune status
☐ 3. Risk for fluid volume deficit related to dehydration
☐ 4. Risk for fetal injury related to uteroplacental insufficiency

CORRECT ANSWER: 2
Infection at any time is a problem for the AIDS client because the immune system is depressed. Invasive procedures, which always increase the risk of infection, are numerous during labor and delivery. Option 1: AIDS clients usually die from opportunistic diseases, not childbirth itself. Option 3: Fluid volume deficit is not a major concern to the nurse at this time. Option 4: The fetus may acquire AIDS in utero, but it is not currently believed that AIDS directly affects the placenta or oxygen transfer to the fetus.

NP: Planning
CN: Safe and effective care environment
CNS: Safety and infection control
CL: Analysis

---

9 A Type 1 diabetic is pregnant for the second time. Her previous pregnancy ended in spontaneous abortion at 18 weeks' gestation. She is now at 22 weeks' gestation. The nurse is responsible for teaching the client about exercise during her pregnancy. Which of the following statements indicates that the client has an appropriate understanding of her exercise needs?

☐ 1. "I know I need to walk with a friend or family member."
☐ 2. "I know I need to vary the times of day when I exercise."
☐ 3. "I know I need to exercise before meals."
☐ 4. "I know I need to drink fluids while I walk."

CORRECT ANSWER: 1
A Type 1 diabetic may become hypoglycemic while exercising. Someone must accompany her for her safety. Option 2: She should exercise at the same time each day. Option 3: She needs to exercise after meals, when blood sugar is high. Option 4: Fluids are not necessary, but the client needs to bring a simple carbohydrate with her to treat hypoglycemia.

NP: Evaluation
CN: Physiological integrity
CNS: Reduction of risk potential
CL: Application

10 A 23-year-old primigravida delivers a healthy 6-lb, 13-oz boy by vaginal delivery. During an assessment the next day, the nurse is examining her lower extremities for signs and symptoms of thrombophlebitis. Which of the following is the best sign to assess?

- ☐ 1. Chadwick's sign
- ☐ 2. Hegar's sign
- ☐ 3. Homans' sign
- ☐ 4. Goodell's sign

CORRECT ANSWER: 3

Assessment of Homans' sign is accomplished by asking the client to stretch her legs out with her knees slightly flexed. The nurse grasps and dorsiflexes the foot. Pain or discomfort at the back of the knee or calf during this manipulation suggests thrombophlebitis. Options 1, 2, and 4 are observable or palpable changes in the cervix, vagina, or uterus that indicate pregnancy.

NP: Assessment
CN: Physiological integrity
CNS: Reduction of risk potential
CL: Comprehension

---

11 A 17-year-old gravida 2, para 1 at 38 weeks' gestation comes to the clinic complaining of headache. She has had leg edema for the past 3 weeks. Her blood pressure is 150/100 mm Hg. The client is admitted for treatment of PIH, and magnesium sulfate I.V. therapy is initiated. The client says she feels "doped and sleepy" and "doesn't like feeling this way." What is the nurse's best response?

- ☐ 1. "That just means the medicine is doing what it's supposed to be doing."
- ☐ 2. "Don't worry; everybody feels like this after taking magnesium sulfate."
- ☐ 3. "That doesn't seem right. I will call the physician and see what he says about it."
- ☐ 4. "This is one side effect of magnesium sulfate therapy; the feeling will go away when the medication is discontinued."

CORRECT ANSWER: 4

Magnesium sulfate acts as a central nervous system (CNS) depressant, so lethargy is a common side effect. Options 1 and 2 provide incomplete information to the client. Option 3 might be appropriate if the nurse found evidence of toxicity (flushing, reflex depression, decreased urine output, or depressed respiration).

NP: Implementation
CN: Physiological integrity
CNS: Pharmacological and parenteral therapies
CL: Application

12 A 38-year-old gravida 4, para 3 at 36 weeks' gestation is admitted with thrombophlebitis. An I.V. heparin drip has been started. The client is on strict bed rest, with the nurse checking vital signs every 4 hours and fetal heart tones every 8 hours. The client is concerned about the effect the drug might have on her baby. She states, "If it makes my blood thinner, then won't it make my baby's blood change?" What is the nurse's most appropriate response?

☐ 1. "Your doctor can answer this for you. Wait until he comes tomorrow and ask him."
☐ 2. "It is impossible for this drug to change your baby's blood."
☐ 3. "Heparin does not cross the placenta, so it cannot get into the baby's blood system."
☐ 4. "The heparin molecule is too large to get to the baby, so it cannot damage the baby."

CORRECT ANSWER: 3
Because its molecular weight is too high, heparin does not cross the placenta and thus would not affect fetal blood. Option 1: The client's concern is urgent. She doesn't need to wait until tomorrow when the nurse can give her a simple explanation now. Option 2: This vague answer does not explain why the heparin will not affect the baby. Option 4: Use of the word "damage" may frighten the client, especially because the response does not exclude the client from injury.

NP: Implementation
CN: Physiological integrity
CNS: Pharmacological and parenteral therapies
CL: Application

---

13 A pregnant client is receiving heparin. Which of the following should be a part of nursing assessment on every shift?

☐ 1. Change in fetal activity and position
☐ 2. Increase in blood pressure and temperature
☐ 3. Any signs of preterm labor and bleeding from an orifice
☐ 4. Homans' sign or periorbital edema

CORRECT ANSWER: 3
Potential complications of heparin therapy are preterm labor and maternal hemorrhage. Option 1: Assessment of fetal activity is important, but fetal position is not significant at this time. Option 2: These are not complications of heparin therapy. Option 4: The client should be assessed for Homans' sign if she is at risk for deep vein thrombosis; periorbital edema is assessed in PIH.

NP: Assessment
CN: Physiological integrity
CNS: Pharmacological and parenteral therapies
CL: Application

14 A 15-year-old primigravida gave birth 2 days ago. She tells her primary nurse that having her own little baby will be wonderful. Which nursing response would best evaluate the accuracy of the client's expectations?

☐ 1. "Tell me what your day will be like after you take your baby home."
☐ 2. "Will anyone be available to help you at home with the baby?"
☐ 3. "Have you had any experience taking care of babies?"
☐ 4. "What are you planning to do with your baby when you return to school?"

CORRECT ANSWER: 1

Teenage lifestyles and support systems can vary immensely. This open-ended question will best help the health team gather data about the teen mother's feelings and expectations. Options 2, 3, and 4 are not open-ended and do not clearly ask the client about her expectations.

NP: Implementation
CN: Health promotion and maintenance
CNS: Growth and development through the life span
CL: Application

---

15 A client notices that her newborn's eyes appear to be crossed. She anxiously points this out to the nurse. What is the nurse's best response?

☐ 1. "This is a temporary condition caused by immature neuromuscular control of the eye muscles."
☐ 2. "Don't worry; it will go away."
☐ 3. "You should call it to the attention of your pediatrician."
☐ 4. "We may have to call in an eye specialist."

CORRECT ANSWER: 1

This provides specific information to promote the client's understanding of newborn characteristics. Option 2 gives false reassurance and is a nontherapeutic effort to reduce the mother's concern. Options 3 and 4 are not needed; the condition is normal and will gradually resolve itself as the eye muscles strengthen over the next 3 to 4 months.

NP: Analysis
CN: Health promotion and maintenance
CNS: Growth and development through the life span
CL: Analysis

---

16 The nurse assesses a newborn's respiratory rate at 46 breaths/minute after 6 hours of life. Respirations are shallow, with periods of apnea lasting up to 5 seconds. Which action should the nurse take next?

☐ 1. Attach an apnea monitor.
☐ 2. Continue routine monitoring.
☐ 3. Follow respiratory arrest protocol.
☐ 4. Call the pediatrician immediately to report findings.

CORRECT ANSWER: 2

Normal respiratory rate is 30 to 60 breaths/minute. Options 1, 3, and 4 are not needed; the listed findings are normal respiratory patterns in newborns.

NP: Implementation
CN: Health promotion and maintenance
CNS: Growth and development through the life span
CL: Application

17 A pale, thin 15-year-old comes to the clinic for a pregnancy test, which is positive. The client states that she and her boyfriend have run away from home and that both are unemployed. Which of the following statements by the nurse would be most therapeutic in beginning the assessment and establishing a relationship based on trust?

- ☐ 1. "How does your mother feel about your situation?"
- ☐ 2. "Have you talked to your mother?"
- ☐ 3. "Sometimes young women find it hard to talk about this with their mothers."
- ☐ 4. "You don't have to tell your mother. What are you going to do?"

CORRECT ANSWER: 3

This response may encourage the client to explore her feelings with a nurse who seems to understand. Options 1 and 4 might elicit some information, but they make assumptions about the client's situation in a way that seems likely to limit further communication or trust. Option 2 is a closed question. Even if the response is "yes," the adolescent may have given the answer she thinks the nurse wants to hear rather than telling the truth.

NP: Assessment
CN: Psychosocial integrity
CNS: Coping and adaptation
CL: Application

---

18 A 19-year-old primigravida is being treated for her second case of simple vaginitis during pregnancy. Which of the following instructions is most important for the nurse to focus on during client teaching?

- ☐ 1. Increase the pH of the vagina by douching regularly.
- ☐ 2. Douche daily with a mild soap solution.
- ☐ 3. Maintain cleanliness and avoid contamination after elimination.
- ☐ 4. Report any signs and symptoms immediately.

CORRECT ANSWER: 3

Simple vaginitis can result from poor hygiene, tight clothing, or emotional stress. Teaching the client proper hygienic measures could help prevent a recurrence. Douching (Options 1 and 2) is not recommended during pregnancy. In any case, the client would want to decrease vaginal pH to support the Döderlein's bacilli, the main defense of the vagina. If douching were ordered, the pH would be lowered by using a weak acid solution (such as vinegar and water), not a soap solution. Option 4 would not help prevent a recurrence.

NP: Implementation
CN: Health promotion and maintenance
CNS: Prevention and early detection of disease
CL: Application

19 A client in her 36th week of pregnancy is admitted to the hospital with vaginal bleeding. After undergoing an ultrasonic scan, she is diagnosed with placenta previa. Which assessment finding would best confirm this diagnosis?

- ☐ 1. A rigid abdomen
- ☐ 2. A soft, nontender uterus
- ☐ 3. Painful vaginal bleeding
- ☐ 4. Hypotension

CORRECT ANSWER: 2

A soft, relaxed, nontender uterus accompanied by vaginal bleeding indicates placenta previa. Option 1: A rigid abdomen indicates abruptio placentae, in which a normally implanted placenta in the upper uterine segment prematurely separates from its implantation site. Option 3: In placenta previa, the placenta is not normally implanted, and the client should not feel pain when it begins to break away. Option 4: Hypotension may indicate many conditions other than placenta previa. Also, bleeding with placenta previa may not be severe enough to cause hypotension.

NP: Assessment
CN: Physiological integrity
CNS: Reduction of risk potential
CL: Application

---

20 A primigravida client is 16 weeks pregnant. Which client teaching instruction would be most important to prevent toxoplasmosis?

- ☐ 1. Cook meats thoroughly.
- ☐ 2. Keep dogs outside.
- ☐ 3. Wash and cook all vegetables.
- ☐ 4. Have antibody titers drawn on a routine basis.

CORRECT ANSWER: 1

Undercooked fresh meats that contain cysts with toxoplasmosis can cause infection. Option 2: Cats, not dogs, carry toxoplasmosis. Option 3: Toxoplasmosis is not carried on vegetables. Option 4: Antibody titers will not prevent toxoplasmosis.

NP: Implementation
CN: Health promotion and maintenance
CNS: Prevention and early detection of disease
CL: Application

---

21 A client is 6 weeks pregnant with her first baby. This is her first prenatal visit. She says to the nurse, "I just can't believe I'm really pregnant. I hope this baby is a good idea." What would be the most likely evaluation the nurse would make from the client's statement?

- ☐ 1. The client is afraid of pregnancy and birth.
- ☐ 2. The client should have waited until she was committed to having a baby.
- ☐ 3. The client is experiencing normal ambivalence about being pregnant.
- ☐ 4. The client may have problems attaching to the baby after birth.

CORRECT ANSWER: 3

Ambivalence is normal in the first trimester of pregnancy, even when a pregnancy is planned and desired. Options 1 and 4 are not substantiated by the evidence supplied. Option 2 is judgmental.

NP: Assessment
CN: Health promotion and maintenance
CNS: Growth and development through the life span
CL: Analysis

22 A client is 22 weeks pregnant with her first baby. Her weight gain is normal, but she complains of constipation. What is the most effective recommendation the nurse can make?

☐ 1. Take a mild laxative daily.
☐ 2. Increase intake of fluids and high-fiber foods.
☐ 3. Relax when trying to move the bowels.
☐ 4. Start a strenuous exercise program.

CORRECT ANSWER: 2

Increased fluids and fiber will soften the stool, making it easier to pass without medication use. Option 1 relies on medication. Option 3 is important but does not address the problem as effectively as increasing fluids and fiber. Option 4 is discouraged during pregnancy unless the client is already accustomed to it. Mild exercise is safe, however, and may increase peristalsis and enhance stool passage.

NP: Implementation
CN: Health promotion and maintenance
CNS: Growth and development through the life span
CL: Application

---

23 A Type 1 diabetic client is gravida 2, para 0, abortus 1. She is now at 37 weeks' gestation. Several tests to determine fetal lung maturity have been performed by amniocentesis. Which of the following is the most reliable indicator of fetal lung maturity?

☐ 1. Lecithin/sphingomyelin (L/S) ratio of 2:1
☐ 2. The presence of phosphatidylglycerol
☐ 3. Increasing bilirubin levels
☐ 4. Decreasing estriol levels

CORRECT ANSWER: 2

The presence of phosphatidylglycerol is a reliable sign that the lungs are mature. Option 1: The L/S ratio must be higher in the diabetic because high insulin levels inhibit surfactant production. Option 3: Bilirubin levels do not measure fetal lung maturity and should decrease at term; increasing levels may signal a fetal blood incompatibility. Option 4: Estriol levels do not measure fetal lung maturity.

NP: Assessment
CN: Health promotion and maintenance
CNS: Growth and development through the life span
CL: Application

24 A client in her 7th month of pregnancy has been complaining of back pain and wants to know what can be done to relieve it. Which of the following responses by the nurse is most effective?

☐ 1. "You need to lie down more during the day to get off your feet."
☐ 2. "Avoid lifting heavy loads, and try using the pelvic tilt exercise."
☐ 3. "Have others pick things up for you so you don't have to bend over so much."
☐ 4. "Your back pain will go away after the baby is born."

CORRECT ANSWER: 2

The pelvic tilt exercise, which can be done standing as well as lying down, can greatly relieve back discomfort. As the pregnancy progresses into the last trimester, women typically develop a "swayback" curvature of the spine to counterbalance the enlarging fetus. Tilting of the pelvis aligns the spine, decreasing pressure and back discomfort. Option 1 may not be possible or convenient for some clients. Also, the supine position may not be comfortable for some clients and may cause vena cava syndrome (dizziness on rising and decreased circulation to the fetus). Option 3 may not be realistic for the client's circumstances, nor does it address back pain as effectively as the pelvic tilt. Option 4 does not relieve the client's discomfort.

NP: Implementation
CN: Health promotion and maintenance
CNS: Growth and development through the life span
CL: Application

---

25 A nurse instructs a prenatal class about the importance of doing Kegel exercises frequently. Kegel exercises are effective for which of the following?

☐ 1. To promote better breathing by strengthening the diaphragm muscle
☐ 2. To help maintain good perineal muscle tone by tightening the pubococcygeus muscle
☐ 3. To minimize leg cramps by strengthening the calf muscles
☐ 4. To prepare the mother for pushing by strengthening the abdominal muscles

CORRECT ANSWER: 2

Kegel exercises are performed by alternately tightening and releasing perineal muscles to strengthen the pubococcygeus muscle and increase its elasticity. The pubococcygeus muscle supports internal organs, such as the uterus and bladder. Options 1, 3, and 4: Kegel exercises do not affect breathing or muscles of the diaphragm, leg, or abdomen.

NP: Planning
CN: Health promotion and maintenance
CNS: Prevention and early detection of disease
CL: Application

26 A 21-year-old primigravida has an emergency cesarean delivery under general anesthesia because of unanticipated fetal distress. One postoperative intervention is to assist her to turn every 2 hours. Which of the following conditions is this intervention intended to prevent?

☐ 1. Pressure ulcers
☐ 2. Muscular stiffness
☐ 3. Respiratory complications
☐ 4. Venous stasis

CORRECT ANSWER: 3
General anesthesia and postoperative pain may lead to immobility, which predisposes to respiratory complications postoperatively. Changing positions, along with coughing and deep breathing, is done to prevent respiratory complications. Option 1: It is unlikely that an otherwise healthy young woman would develop pressure ulcers during a brief postoperative period. Option 2: Muscular stiffness would, of course, be decreased with frequent turning, but this is not the most important rationale for turning. Option 4: Turning may also decrease venous stasis, but a more effective intervention to decrease venous stasis in the early postoperative period would be leg exercises.

NP: Planning
CN: Physiological integrity
CNS: Reduction of risk potential
CL: Application

---

27 As part of a prenatal nutritional teaching program for a 17-year-old who is concerned about weight gain, which of the following statements by the nurse would be most accurate?

☐ 1. "If you stay away from fast foods, your weight gain will be minimal."
☐ 2. "You're young. You will be able to lose the weight after the baby is born with no problems."
☐ 3. "During pregnancy a woman's caloric needs increase by about 300 calories per day. If you like, I can help you with some meal planning."
☐ 4. "Keep your caloric intake to around 1,000 calories per day. In this way you will gain only the proper amount of weight."

CORRECT ANSWER: 3
This answer supplies the client with facts and offers help and guidance for a healthier pregnancy. Options 1 and 2 are unrealistic and offer false reassurance. Option 4 is insufficient to nourish a teenage girl and the growing fetus.

NP: Planning
CN: Health promotion and maintenance
CNS: Growth and development through the life span
CL: Application

28 A 34-year-old at 32 weeks' gestation tells the nurse that her baby will be sick because she saw a dead dog on the road yesterday. What is the best response by the nurse?

☐ 1. "Your baby will be fine. That's just superstition."
☐ 2. "Don't worry. We'll make sure your baby will be OK."
☐ 3. "I can see that you are concerned. Let's talk about what is bothering you."
☐ 4. "Perhaps so. Your baby should be seen by a physician as soon as it's born."

Correct answer: 3
Some cultures hold that if a pregnant woman looks upon a dead animal, the fetus is exposed to the realm of the dead and may later become ill as a baby. The nurse's response is sensitive to the mother's beliefs and eases the way for the mother to begin to talk about her concern. Option 1 discounts the mother's beliefs. Option 2 dismisses the mother's concerns and offers false reassurance. Option 4 carries empathy over into false validation and overreaction, yet it fails to set up any dialogue with the client.

NP: Implementation
CN: Psychosocial integrity
CNS: Coping and adaptation
CL: Analysis

---

29 Which of the following complications of pregnancy are most common among adolescents?

☐ 1. PIH and iron-deficiency anemia
☐ 2. Hypothyroidism and obesity
☐ 3. Diabetes and cardiac disease
☐ 4. Iron-deficiency anemia and Rh disease

Correct answer: 1
PIH is the most prevalent medical complication in adolescents. This may be related to parity rather than age, however. Most pregnant adolescents are nulliparous, and nulliparity has been determined as an important factor related to PIH. Many adolescents have iron-deficiency anemia even before beginning their pregnancy because of their previous rapid growth spurt. Options 2 and 3 are not specific to adolescent pregnancy. Option 4: Iron-deficiency anemia can be a problem in adolescent pregnancy, but Rh disease has nothing to do with adolescence.

NP: Assessment
CN: Physiological adaptation
CNS: Reduction of risk potential
CL: Comprehension

---

30 The human embryo grows at a very rapid rate. At what gestational age does a single-chambered heart begin to beat and pump its own blood cells through main blood vessels?

☐ 1. Approximately 8 weeks
☐ 2. Approximately 60 days
☐ 3. Approximately 5 weeks
☐ 4. Approximately 24 days

Correct answer: 4
In the embryo's third week, the heart becomes the most advanced organ. Around the 24th day, a single-chambered heart forms just outside the embryo's body cavity and begins beating a regular rhythm, pushing its own primitive blood cells through the main blood vessels. Options 1, 2, and 3: Development has occurred before these times.

NP: Assessment
CN: Health promotion and maintenance
CNS: Growth and development through the life span
CL: Comprehension

31 A 22-year-old client presents to the maternity clinic for her first prenatal visit. She is gravida 1; approximate gestational age is 10 weeks. What is the simplest and most cost-effective means of determining nutritional status?

☐ 1. Food frequency questionnaire and blood tests
☐ 2. Interview focusing on food allergies and intolerances
☐ 3. Anthropometric measures and 24-hour recall
☐ 4. Diet history interview

CORRECT ANSWER: 3

A combination of anthropometric measurements and 24-hour recall provides information about the nutritional status and food choices that can be evaluated immediately and also serves as a starting point for nutrition counseling. Option 1: A food frequency questionnaire might be useful for long-term monitoring after a problem is identified. Option 2: Food allergies and intolerances are only a small part of the nutritional status profile. Option 4: A complex diet history interview requires a highly trained nutritionist and is too costly for general practice.

NP: Assessment
CN: Health promotion and maintenance
CNS: Prevention and early detection of disease
CL: Application

---

32 A 2-week postpartum client inquires about alcohol use during lactation. She tells the nurse she has heard that a small glass of wine or beer before nursing will increase her milk supply and be good for the baby. What is the nurse's best response?

☐ 1. "It is true that a little alcohol before breast-feeding will help your milk supply because it will help you relax."
☐ 2. "Research has shown that it actually decreases the amount of milk the baby will get, perhaps because it affects the taste of your milk."
☐ 3. "A little alcohol will help you to relax and the small amount that will pass through the milk may just help the baby relax."
☐ 4. "You should not even consider drinking alcohol while you are nursing a baby."

CORRECT ANSWER: 2

According to several recent studies, breast-fed babies consume less milk on days when their mothers drink alcohol. Options 1 and 3: In light of the recent studies and the incidence of alcohol-related problems in our society, encouraging alcohol use by breast-feeding mothers seems unwise. Option 4: This judgmental response negates the responsible behavior that the client demonstrated by asking a nurse for advice.

NP: Implementation
CN: Health promotion and maintenance
CNS: Prevention and early detection of disease
CL: Analysis

33 A client in the first trimester complains of nausea every morning and asks about medicine to prevent it. What is the nurse's most helpful response?

☐ 1. "Let me tell you about some methods to control nausea without medication."
☐ 2. "You shouldn't take medication during pregnancy, especially during the early weeks."
☐ 3. "I'll ask the physician if you can have something."
☐ 4. "You'll probably have a lot less nausea in just a few weeks."

CORRECT ANSWER: 1
This gives concrete help to the client without involving drug therapy. Options 2 and 4 may be true in general, but they don't give any help to the woman. They may be used as adjunct explanations along with the nurse's specific suggestions. Option 3 (drug therapy) is inappropriate without evidence that the nausea is detrimental to the client's health.

NP: Implementation
CN: Health promotion and maintenance
CNS: Growth and development through the life span
CL: Application

---

34 A client is in the second trimester of her first pregnancy. She confides that she has been smoking about half a pack of cigarettes per day because she had been told that smoking results in smaller babies and she is fearful of delivery. What is the best response by the nurse?

☐ 1. "You should know better than to smoke at all. Your baby will be much better off if it is bigger."
☐ 2. "I can understand your concern. A few cigarettes should not hurt the baby."
☐ 3. "Unfortunately, the smaller size of the baby of a smoking mother has more to do with its overall development than with the ease of delivery. Let's talk about it."
☐ 4. "Unfortunately, that is just not true. Your baby's size is determined by factors unrelated to smoking."

CORRECT ANSWER: 3
The truth is that smoking does affect the size of the baby — including the size of its brain. Option 1: This judgmental answer does not enhance further communication about two important issues, smoking and the fear of delivery. Option 2: This gives false reassurance; research has clearly shown cigarette smoking to be harmful to the developing fetus. Option 4: Smoking can cause lower birth weight and intrauterine growth retardation (IUGR).

NP: Assessment
CN: Health promotion and maintenance
CNS: Prevention and early detection of disease
CL: Analysis

---

35 While evaluating the needs of a client during the second trimester, the nurse can anticipate which of the following?

☐ 1. Feelings of disbelief and ambivalence
☐ 2. A feeling of clumsiness and "ugliness"
☐ 3. Increasing introspection but a general sense of well-being
☐ 4. Anxiety about the labor and delivery experience

CORRECT ANSWER: 3
Women generally feel best during the second trimester. Most enjoy a rather tranquil few months when they experience quickening and begin to "show" without the heaviness and awkwardness of the third trimester. Option 1 is more common in the first trimester; Options 2 and 4, in the third trimester.

NP: Assessment
CN: Health promotion and maintenance
CNS: Growth and development through the life span
CL: Comprehension

36 A primipara client in her 10th week of pregnancy calls the nurse to say that she is experiencing slight vaginal bleeding. What is the nurse's best response?

☐ 1. "Lie down on your left side and call again if the bleeding worsens."
☐ 2. "Save any perineal pads, clots, and tissue and come to the clinic right away."
☐ 3. "Avoid sexual intercourse for the next 2 weeks."
☐ 4. "Continue your normal activities and increase your fluid intake."

CORRECT ANSWER: 2
Vaginal bleeding, a sign of threatened abortion, warrants immediate attention. Saving perineal pads and any matter passed vaginally will make evaluation more reliable. Option 1: The left lateral position is important during the last trimester, when the possibility of vena cava syndrome exists. Option 3: Sexual activity is not usually implicated in spontaneous abortion. Option 4: These actions fail to address the client's need to see the physician immediately.
NP: Planning
CN: Physiological integrity
CNS: Physiological adaptation
CL: Analysis

---

37 A pregnant client is taking folic acid. During prenatal teaching, which of the following foods would the nurse recommend as high in folic acid?

☐ 1. Egg yolks
☐ 2. Fruit
☐ 3. Bread
☐ 4. Milk

CORRECT ANSWER: 1
Egg yolks, nuts, seeds, and liver are all high in folic acid. Options 2, 3, and 4 are not good sources of folic acid.
NP: Implementation
CN: Health promotion and maintenance
CNS: Prevention and early detection of disease
CL: Application

---

38 A 27-year-old primipara in her 5th month of pregnancy has been receiving regular prenatal care since week 8. She complains of feeling dizzy, breathless, and clammy on rising from bed in the morning. In responding to the client, the nurse would assess for which of the following conditions?

☐ 1. Shock
☐ 2. Hemorrhage
☐ 3. Supine hypotension
☐ 4. Fainting

CORRECT ANSWER: 3
Supine hypotension is a common complication of pregnancy. Option 1: Although some symptoms of shock resemble those seen in supine hypotension, the given data would not predispose the client to shock. Option 2: The assessment data do not indicate hemorrhage. Option 4: The symptoms given in the case study do not describe fainting itself.
NP: Assessment
CN: Physiological integrity
CNS: Reduction of risk potential
CL: Application

39 In assessing a client for pregnancy, the nurse would look for which positive sign?

- ☐ 1. Quickening
- ☐ 2. Amenorrhea
- ☐ 3. Fetal movement felt by the examiner
- ☐ 4. Enlarging uterus

Correct answer: 3

Fetal movement detected by an examiner is an objective, positive sign of pregnancy. Quickening (Option 1), a subjective sign of pregnancy experienced by the woman, is not as reliable as an independent assessment. Amenorrhea (Option 2) and enlargement of the uterus (Option 4) can occur in a molar pregnancy or for various reasons unrelated to pregnancy.

NP: Assessment
CN: Health promotion and maintenance
CNS: Growth and development through the life span
CL: Application

---

40 A 35-year-old client is in the 8th month of her first pregnancy. Her physician orders a biophysical profile to be conducted the next day. What equipment would the nurse assemble to conduct this test?

- ☐ 1. Sphygmomanometer and thermometer
- ☐ 2. Ultrasound machine and fetal monitor
- ☐ 3. Ultrasound machine and sphygmomanometer
- ☐ 4. Fetal monitor and electronic blood pressure measuring device

Correct answer: 2

During a biophysical profile, the amount and quality of fetal movement and the amount of amniotic fluid are measured via ultrasonography followed by a nonstress test. Options 1, 3, and 4 do not list the correct equipment for this profile.

NP: Implementation
CN: Health promotion and maintenance
CNS: Growth and development through the life span
CL: Application

---

41 A 23-year-old primigravida client has a normal vaginal delivery. The next day, the nurse assesses the client's lochia for color, amount, and the presence of clots. Which of the following best describes lochia on the first postpartum day?

- ☐ 1. Dark red (lochia rubra), large amount, with many clots
- ☐ 2. Pink (lochia serosa), moderate amount, no clots
- ☐ 3. White (lochia alba), scant amount, no clots
- ☐ 4. Dark red (lochia rubra), moderate amount, with a few small clots

Correct answer: 4

Lochia rubra is usually seen during the first 1 to 3 days. It should be moderate in amount and may include some small clots. Four to eight perineal pads are used daily on average. Option 1: Heavy bleeding could be from uterine atony or retained placental fragments and therefore requires further investigation. Option 2: Lochia serosa follows lochia rubra and lasts to about the 10th postpartum day. Option 3: Lochia alba is seen from approximately the 11th to the 21st postpartum day.

NP: Assessment
CN: Health promotion and maintenance
CNS: Growth and development through the life span
CL: Comprehension

42 A baby born at 34 weeks' gestation has a surfactant deficit. Which of the following conditions would the nurse most likely find in completing a newborn assessment?

☐ 1. Jaundice
☐ 2. Sternal retractions
☐ 3. Abdominal distention
☐ 4. Frothy, blood-tinged sputum

CORRECT ANSWER: 2

A surfactant deficit reduces lung compliance and increases the inspiratory pressure needed to expand the lungs. It does not affect the liver (Option 1) or abdomen (Option 3). Frothy, blood-tinged sputum (Option 4) is more closely associated with pulmonary edema.

NP: Assessment
CN: Physiological integrity
CNS: Physiological adaptation
CL: Application

---

43 A client has a boggy uterus during Stage IV of her delivery. Four hours postpartum, the nurse is preparing to administer methylergonovine maleate (Methergine) 0.2 mg P.O. as prescribed every 6 hours. The client's vital signs are: temperature, 100.4°F; pulse, 60 beats/minute; respirations, 14 breaths/minute; blood pressure, 140/90 mm Hg. Which is the most appropriate intervention?

☐ 1. Administer the drug STAT.
☐ 2. Administer the drug and call the physician.
☐ 3. Administer the drug and recheck vital signs.
☐ 4. Do not administer the drug.

CORRECT ANSWER: 4

Methylergonovine maleate, a vasoconstrictor, can cause hypertension. It should not be administered to a hypertensive client.

NP: Application
CN: Physiological integrity
CNS: Pharmacological and parenteral therapies
CL: Analysis

---

44 A multigravida in her 34th week of gestation presents in the emergency department complaining of vaginal bleeding. Which of the following should be the nurse's first action?

☐ 1. Establish I.V. access.
☐ 2. Assess fetal heart rate (FHR) and maternal blood pressure.
☐ 3. Prepare the client for a cesarean section.
☐ 4. Assess maternal heart rate and respiratory rate.

CORRECT ANSWER: 2

FHR and maternal blood pressure will provide important data on the conditions of mother and fetus. Option 1: An I.V. should be started after the maternal-fetal dyad is assessed. Option 3: Preparing the client for a cesarean delivery before determining the cause of the vaginal bleeding would be premature. Option 4: These assessments, while important, are not the best indicators of maternal health status and provide no information about fetal health.

NP: Implementation
CN: Physiological integrity
CNS: Physiological adaptation
CL: Analysis

45 A client at term arrives at the labor room experiencing contractions every 4 minutes. After a brief assessment, she is admitted and an electronic fetal monitor (EFM) is applied. Which of the following would alert the nurse to an increased potential for fetal distress?

☐ 1. Weight gain of 30 pounds
☐ 2. Maternal age of 32 years
☐ 3. Blood pressure of 146/90 mm Hg
☐ 4. Treatment for syphilis at 15 weeks' gestation

CORRECT ANSWER: 3
Blood pressure of 146/90 mm Hg indicates PIH. Over time, PIH reduces blood flow to the placenta; it can cause IUGR and other problems that make the fetus less able to tolerate the stress of labor. Option 1: A weight gain of 30 pounds is within the expected parameters for a healthy pregnancy. Option 2: A woman over age 30 does not have a greater risk of complications if her general condition is healthy before pregnancy. Option 4: Syphilis that has been treated does not pose an additional risk.

NP: Assessment
CN: Health promotion and maintenance
CNS: Growth and development through the life span
CL: Application

---

46 During labor, meconium in the amniotic fluid is a normal finding in which of the following situations?

☐ 1. Preterm labor
☐ 2. Cephalopelvic disproportion
☐ 3. Prolonged latent phase
☐ 4. Breech presentation

CORRECT ANSWER: 4
Meconium in a breech presentation may be caused by compression of the fetus's intestinal tract on descent. Options 1, 2, and 3: Meconium in these situations could signify fetal distress caused by a brief period of fetal hypoxia.

NP: Assessment
CN: Physiological integrity
CNS: Reduction of risk potential
CL: Comprehension

---

47 Which of the following indicates fetal distress?

☐ 1. Fetal scalp pH of 7.14
☐ 2. FHR of 144 beats/minute
☐ 3. Acceleration of FHR with contractions
☐ 4. Long-term variability

CORRECT ANSWER: 1
A scalp pH of less than 7.25 indicates acidosis and fetal hypoxia. Options 2, 3, and 4 are normal responses of a healthy fetus to labor.

NP: Assessment
CN: Physiological integrity
CNS: Reduction of risk potential
CL: Comprehension

---

48 A primipara at 32 weeks' gestation comes to the hospital complaining of vaginal bleeding. She has soaked one peripad. She has no pain or cramps. In performing an assessment, the nurse would suspect which of the following?

☐ 1. Placenta previa
☐ 2. Abruptio placentae
☐ 3. Vasa previa
☐ 4. Incompetent cervix

CORRECT ANSWER: 1
Painless vaginal bleeding is the classic sign of placenta previa. Option 2: Abruptio placentae is painful. Option 3: Vasa previa occurs with ruptured membranes. Option 4: An incompetent cervix causes pressure sensations.

NP: Assessment
CN: Physiological integrity
CNS: Physiological adaptation
CL: Application

49 A client at 42 weeks' gestation is 3 cm dilated, 30% effaced, with membranes intact and the fetus at +2 station. FHR is 140 to 150 beats/minute. The client is started on oxytocin (Pitocin) to induce labor. After 2 hours, the nurse notes on the EFM that the FHR has been ranging from 160 to 190 beats/minute for the past 10 minutes. The client states that her baby has been extremely active. Uterine contractions are strong, occurring every 3 to 4 minutes and lasting 40 to 60 seconds. What part of this assessment data would indicate fetal distress?

☐ 1. Uterine contractions lasting 40 to 60 seconds
☐ 2. Strong uterine contractions
☐ 3. Uterine contractions occurring every 3 to 4 minutes
☐ 4. FHR ranging from 160 to 190 beats/minute

CORRECT ANSWER: 4

Fetal tachycardia and excessive fetal activity are the first signs of fetal hypoxia (distress). Option 1: The duration of uterine contractions is within normal limits. Option 2: Uterine intensity can be mild, moderate, or strong. Option 3: The frequency of contractions is within normal limits for the active phase of labor.

NP: Evaluation
CN: Physiological integrity
CNS: Physiological adaptation
CL: Analysis

---

50 Which of the following would be the most likely effect of pregnancy in an adolescent client?

☐ 1. Delayed independence from parents
☐ 2. Development of the maturity to sustain complex interpersonal relationships
☐ 3. Increased motivation to develop financial stability
☐ 4. Increased awareness and use of contraceptives

CORRECT ANSWER: 1

A pregnant adolescent enters a cycle of defeat that strains relationships, disrupts education, and impairs earning power. Pregnancy and child rearing usually force the adolescent into prolonged dependence on the parents for support and assistance. Option 2: Pregnancy and child rearing can delay adolescent development and interfere with the formation of stable relationships. Option 3: Financial independence proves difficult to achieve for adolescent parents, many of whom never complete their education. Option 4: One teenage pregnancy commonly is followed by another, especially if the first one occurred in younger adolescence.

NP: Assessment
CN: Health promotion and maintenance
CNS: Growth and development through the life span
CL: Analysis

51 A client is admitted to the labor and delivery unit in active labor. She has had no prenatal care but appears to be between 32 and 35 weeks' gestation. History reveals that she is gravida 5, para 1, abortus 3. She tells the nurse she thinks her friend gave her a cigarette containing crack cocaine. What should the nurse do next?

- ☐ 1. Move the precipitant delivery cart to the labor room, and notify the neonatologist on call.
- ☐ 2. Teach the mother controlled breathing techniques.
- ☐ 3. Call a family member to come to the hospital.
- ☐ 4. Call the friend who gave the client the cigarette and find out exactly what the drug was.

CORRECT ANSWER: 1

Cocaine causes increased uterine contractility, preterm labor, and illness in babies born to addicted mothers. This client is in active labor, has a questionable history, and an undetermined length of gestation. The nurse should anticipate a quick delivery and a small, sick baby. Option 2: This client is not in a teachable frame of mind or situation. Option 3: Calling a family member is not a priority when a high-risk birth is imminent. Option 4: The client's friend may be impossible to locate and may not know exactly what was in the cigarette.

NP: Implementation
CN: Physiological integrity
CNS: Physiological adaptation
CL: Application

---

52 A client at 32 weeks' gestation who is leaking amniotic fluid is placed on an EFM. The nurse interprets the monitor strip to indicate uterine irritability, with contractions occurring every 4 to 6 minutes. The physician orders subcutaneous terbutaline (Brethine). Which of the following teaching statements is appropriate for this client?

- ☐ 1. "This medicine will make you breathe better."
- ☐ 2. "You will probably feel no different than if you had taken a Tylenol."
- ☐ 3. "You may feel a fluttering or tight sensation in your chest."
- ☐ 4. "This will make your mouth feel dry and make you thirsty."

CORRECT ANSWER: 3

A tight or fluttering sensation in the chest is a common side effect of terbutaline. To counter this effect, the drug is commonly administered with hydroxyzine hydrochloride (Vistaril). Option 1: Terbutaline does relieve bronchospasms, but this is not why the client is receiving it. Option 2: Terbutaline can produce clearly perceived side effects. Option 4: Mouth dryness may occur with the inhaled form of terbutaline but is unlikely with the subcutaneous form.

NP: Implementation
CN: Physiological integrity
CNS: Pharmacological and parenteral therapies
CL: Application

53 A client delivers a 9-lb, 10-oz baby vaginally, with a midline episiotomy. Shortly after delivery, the client complains of not feeling well. In assessing for possible uterine hemorrhage, the nurse should note which of the following?

☐ 1. Severe cramping, chills, and shaking
☐ 2. Extreme fatigue and lethargy
☐ 3. Cool, clammy, pale skin and anxiety
☐ 4. Hunger, thirst, and hot flashes

CORRECT ANSWER: 3
These signs of impending hypovolemic shock require immediate assessment of lochia, fundus tone, and vital signs. Options 1 and 2: These symptoms are normal for the recovery phase. Option 4: Hunger and thirst are common in mothers who have a normal vaginal delivery without heavy sedation. Hot flashes commonly occur several hours postpartum and are brought about by hormonal changes.
NP: Assessment
CN: Physiological integrity
CNS: Physiological adaptation
CL: Analysis

---

54 A 31-year-old primigravida has had an uncomplicated pregnancy. At 41 weeks' gestation, she is admitted to the labor suite for oxytocin induction of labor. The pre-labor evaluation reveals the client's cervix to be 3 cm dilated, 50% effaced, soft, and in anterior position. Fetal station is 0. These assessment data yield a score of 9 in the Bishop scoring system. Based on these findings, what would the nurse expect to take place?

☐ 1. The induction most probably will be successful because the cervix is favorable.
☐ 2. The induction most probably will not be successful because the cervix is not favorable.
☐ 3. The induction should be delayed until the cervix is 75% effaced.
☐ 4. The induction should be delayed until 42 weeks' gestation.

CORRECT ANSWER: 1
A soft cervix in the anterior position, 50% effaced, and dilated at least 2 cm, with the fetal head at +1 station or lower (Bishop score of 9), is favorable for successful induction of labor. Assessment data do not indicate that induction will not succeed (Option 2) or that it should be delayed (Options 3 and 4).
NP: Assessment
CN: Health promotion and maintenance
CNS: Growth and development through the life span
CL: Analysis

---

55 A 26-year-old primigravida is in labor. Her cervix is 5 cm dilated and 75% effaced; the fetus is at 0 station. The client requests medication to relieve the discomfort of contractions, and the physician prescribes an epidural regional block. What position should the nurse help the client to assume when the epidural is administered?

☐ 1. Lithotomy
☐ 2. Supine
☐ 3. Prone
☐ 4. Lateral

CORRECT ANSWER: 4
The client is placed on her left side, with shoulders parallel and legs slightly flexed. The epidural space, the potential space between the dura mater and the ligamentum flavum, is readily accessed with the client on her side. None of the other positions allows proper access to the epidural space.
NP: Implementation
CN: Physiological integrity
CNS: Reduction of risk potential
CL: Application

56 A client is in labor with her first baby. Which of the following would indicate that the client has moved into the second stage of labor?

☐ 1. The client has an uncontrollable urge to bear down.

☐ 2. The client has a decrease in bloody show.

☐ 3. The client becomes increasingly talkative.

☐ 4. The client takes three deep cleansing breaths.

CORRECT ANSWER: 1

One sign indicating onset of labor's second stage is the involuntary urge to bear down. This is caused by the Ferguson reflex, which is activated when the presenting part of the fetus approaches or touches the perineal floor. Option 2: The bloody show increases, not decreases, in Stage II labor. Option 3: The client would not become more talkative. She would either be more apprehensive and irritable or be pushing and then resting between contractions. Option 4: Cleansing breaths may be taken any time to increase oxygenation and promote relaxation.

NP: Assessment
CN: Health promotion and maintenance
CNS: Growth and development through the life span
CL: Comprehension

---

57 After assessing the nutritional status of a 21-year-old client at 10 weeks' gestation, the nurse chooses the diagnosis "Knowledge deficit (lack of exposure) related to nutritional needs during pregnancy." What should the nurse include in the plan of care?

☐ 1. Identify learning goals for the client.

☐ 2. Tell the client to establish appropriate learning goals.

☐ 3. Outline the decisions that the client will need to make.

☐ 4. Identify factors that may affect the client's learning.

CORRECT ANSWER: 4

This involves establishing a baseline that will be more likely to result in relevant and appropriate learning. Options 1, 2, and 3 fail to include the client in the planning.

NP: Planning
CN: Health promotion and maintenance
CNS: Growth and development through the life span
CL: Analysis

58 A nurse is reviewing prenatal care with a client. Which of the following statements by the client best expresses adequate understanding of nutritional needs during pregnancy?

☐ 1. "I expect to gain a few pounds each month at first. Then I will really get big and put on 20 pounds or so."

☐ 2. "I guess I will get big and gain 20 to 30 pounds and look pregnant."

☐ 3. "Since I have to eat for two, I should eat whatever I want whenever I feel hungry."

☐ 4. "I will need to eat more so that I will gain about 25 pounds, but I want to make sure I don't fill up with junk food."

CORRECT ANSWER: 4

This statement shows an understanding of nutritional needs during pregnancy. Option 1 accurately portrays weight gain but does not express an understanding of nutritional needs. Option 2 does not show an understanding of either nutritional needs or how and when the weight gain will occur. Option 3 is a common rationalization that can result in excessive weight gain.

NP: Evaluation
CN: Health promotion and maintenance
CNS: Growth and development through the life span
CL: Analysis

---

59 A client in active labor is having difficulty remaining focused. Her husband, sister, and mother are in the room with her. The fetal monitor shows slowing of the FHR that begins after the peak of each contraction. Which of the following nursing measures is best for the client?

☐ 1. Have the client get up and walk for a while.

☐ 2. Have the client lie on her left side, and ask the family to take turns being with the client one at a time.

☐ 3. Leave the client and the family alone.

☐ 4. Turn on the television to give the client something to focus on.

CORRECT ANSWER: 2

FHR can slow for various reasons, including decreased maternal blood flow to the uterus. Turning onto the left side promotes effective blood flow by relieving pressure from the great vessels that run down the back to the legs and feed the uterus. Limiting the client to one visitor at a time will cause fewer distractions and improve her chances of focusing properly on breathing techniques. Option 1: The client cannot walk at this stage of labor. Option 3: Intervention is appropriate at this time. Option 4: Turning on the television would increase the stimuli and make focusing even more difficult for the client.

NP: Implementation
CN: Health promotion and maintenance
CNS: Growth and development through the life span
CL: Application

60 A 15-year-old pregnant client comes alone to the maternity clinic and states that she and her boyfriend have run away from home. Neither is employed. Which of the following goals is likely to have the greatest long-term effect on the future well-being of this client?

- ☐ 1. Promotion of self-esteem
- ☐ 2. Promotion of physical well-being
- ☐ 3. Promotion of family adaptation
- ☐ 4. Facilitation of prenatal education

Correct answer: 1

Teenage pregnancy commonly is related to problems of indecision, poor self-image, and egocentrism. If the client can develop self-esteem, the other goals may follow, and such problems as child abuse, drug abuse, and unemployment may be overcome or avoided. Options 2, 3, and 4 are important goals but not as far-reaching as the development of self-esteem.

NP: Planning
CN: Psychosocial integrity
CNS: Coping and adaptation
CL: Analysis

---

61 A 17-year-old primigravida with severe PIH has been receiving magnesium sulfate I.V. for 3 hours. The nurse assesses deep tendon reflexes (DTR), vital signs, and fetal heart tones every 15 minutes and urine output hourly. The latest assessment yields the following data: DTR, +1; blood pressure, 150/100 mm Hg; pulse, 92 beats/minute; respiratory rate, 10 breaths/minute; urine output, 20 ml/hour. The client appears flushed and complains of feeling warm. Which nursing action would be most appropriate in light of the current assessment data?

- ☐ 1. Take no action; continue monitoring per standards of care.
- ☐ 2. Discontinue the magnesium sulfate infusion.
- ☐ 3. Increase the infusion rate by 5 gtt/minute.
- ☐ 4. Decrease the infusion rate by 5 gtt/minute.

Correct answer: 2

Magnesium sulfate should be withheld if the client's respiratory rate or urine output falls below specified levels or if reflexes are diminished or absent. Many protocols require discontinuing magnesium sulfate if respirations fall below 12 breaths/minute. Normal DTR is +2; this client's have fallen to +1. Urine output is below the accepted minimum of 25 to 30 ml/hour. The client also shows other signs of impending toxicity, such as flushing and feeling warm. Option 1: Inaction will not resolve the client's suppressed DTR and low respiratory rate and urine output. Option 3: The client is already showing CNS depression because of excessive magnesium sulfate. Option 4: Impending toxicity indicates that the infusion should be discontinued rather than just slowed down.

NP: Evaluation
CN: Physiological integrity
CNS: Pharmacological and parenteral therapies
CL: Application

62 A diabetic client delivers a 6-lb baby at 36 weeks' gestation. The infant is placed in the neonatal intensive care unit (NICU). The mother is grieving over the early delivery. What action by the nurse would be most helpful to the client?

☐ 1. Seek involvement of external support systems to provide emotional comfort and material resources for the client.
☐ 2. Generalize how the client must be feeling based on her written history and pregnancy course.
☐ 3. Encourage the client to immerse herself in her intense feeling of grief.
☐ 4. Call the client's minister to obtain spiritual support for her and her family.

CORRECT ANSWER: 1

Based on their knowledge of the client's unique needs and coping mechanisms, close family and friends can offer support and resources to deal most effectively with the client's concerns. Option 2 does not allow the client to express feelings. Option 3 (expressing grief), although important, does not address the critical need for support systems. Option 4 is one of many support systems covered by Option 1.

NP: Planning
CN: Psychosocial integrity
CNS: Coping and adaptation
CL: Application

---

63 A baby weighed 3,350 grams at birth. On discharge (postpartum day 3), his weight had decreased to 3,100 grams. His mother is upset and asks whether the baby was fed in the nursery. Which of these responses would be most helpful?

☐ 1. "Most newborns lose 10% to 30% of their birth weight."
☐ 2. "I understand your concern. His weight loss is excessive."
☐ 3. "Show me how you have been feeding the baby."
☐ 4. "I can see that you are worried. His weight loss is an expected one. He will probably start to gain weight now."

CORRECT ANSWER: 4

Physiological weight loss of 5% to 10% occurs after birth due to fluid shift. The weight loss in Option 1 is too high. Option 2 is incorrect because this infant's weight loss is within expected percentages. Option 3 implies to the mother that she has been doing something wrong.

NP: Implementation
CN: Health promotion and maintenance
CNS: Growth and development through the life span
CL: Application

---

64 A new mother is discharged 16 hours after delivery. Which of the following symptoms would require the new mother to contact her health care provider?

☐ 1. Vaginal tenderness and dryness during sexual activity
☐ 2. Uterus that is no longer palpable abdominally after 2 weeks
☐ 3. Bright red lochia with an increased flow rate
☐ 4. Fatigue and weight loss

CORRECT ANSWER: 3

New mothers should be aware of complications that can occur after discharge. A change in the color of lochia with increased flow may indicate retained placental fragments. Options 1, 2, and 4 are normal symptoms after delivery; in addition, sexual activity (Option 1) is usually not resumed for several weeks after delivery.

NP: Implementation
CN: Health promotion and maintenance
CNS: Growth and development through the life span
CL: Application

65 A 21-year-old primigravida had an emergency cesarean section because of anticipated fetal distress. Three days after her delivery, the client seems preoccupied and troubled, and the nurse notes her crying in her room after visitors leave. She tells the nurse that her incision is ugly and that she "feels like a failure." In responding to the client, the nurse should consider which of the following?

- ☐ 1. The client is experiencing abnormal feelings and needs psychiatric care.
- ☐ 2. The client is grieving the loss of her anticipated childbirth experience.
- ☐ 3. The client is in the dependent taking-in phase described by Rubin.
- ☐ 4. The client is tired and upset from having too many visitors.

CORRECT ANSWER: 2

Some women who deliver by cesarean section, especially when unexpected, have negative feelings afterward and blame themselves for their inability to deliver "normally." Grieving such a loss of vaginal delivery is normal. Option 1: The client's feelings are not abnormal. Option 3: The taking-in phase occurs in the first day or two. Option 4: There is not enough evidence to indicate that the client was having too many visitors.

NP: Planning
CN: Psychosocial integrity
CNS: Coping and adaptation
CL: Analysis

---

66 A gravida 3 delivered her first child vaginally and her second child by cesarean section due to a complete placenta previa. After consulting with her physician about the third delivery, the client agrees to attempt a vaginal birth after cesarean (VBAC). She presents at the local hospital in early labor, 3 to 4 cm dilated, 80% effaced, at +1 station. The nurse reviewing the client's prenatal record notes that the client had received the appropriate incision to attempt a VBAC. Which type of incision should be listed on her prenatal record?

- ☐ 1. Upper uterine segment classical incision
- ☐ 2. Lower uterine segment vertical incision
- ☐ 3. Combination upper and lower uterine T incision
- ☐ 4. Lower uterine segment transverse incision

CORRECT ANSWER: 4

The lower uterine segment transverse incision has less side to side tension; therefore, dehiscence is rare. This is the only type of uterine incision that allows for a VBAC. Options 1, 2, and 3 include vertical cuts, and the incisions are more likely to rupture with contractions.

NP: Assessment
CN: Physiological integrity
CNS: Reduction of risk potential
CL: Application

67 During her first prenatal visit to the obstetrician's office, a client complains of increased vaginal drainage. Which of the following responses by the nurse is most appropriate?

☐ 1. "This is normal during pregnancy. Just be sure to wash daily with soap and water."
☐ 2. "This may indicate an infection, and the drainage will have to be cultured."
☐ 3. "This is normal during pregnancy, and you can douche daily."
☐ 4. "This is an unusual occurrence, and you must be seen by the physician immediately."

CORRECT ANSWER: 1
Increased vaginal drainage is normal during pregnancy. The client should be instructed on proper perineum care and told not to douche during pregnancy. Options 2 and 4 incorrectly suggest that the increased drainage is abnormal. Option 3 inappropriately instructs the client to douche daily.

NP: Implementation
CN: Health promotion and maintenance
CNS: Growth and development through the life span
CL: Application

---

68 A 19-year-old primigravida is admitted to the labor and delivery unit in labor. She is 2 cm dilated and 50% effaced, and the fetal head is at 0 station. She is having moderately strong 40-second contractions every 5 minutes. She seems rather anxious and becomes very tense during each contraction. When the client asks for pain relief, what should the nurse do next?

☐ 1. Determine the source of her anxiety and institute interventions to help her relax.
☐ 2. Immediately check the physician's order and give her the analgesic ordered.
☐ 3. Inform her that the baby's head is not down far enough just yet, but that as soon as it is, medication will be given.
☐ 4. Tell her that her contractions are only moderately strong, and that she should wait until later to take medication.

CORRECT ANSWER: 1
Decreasing anxiety can break the fear-tension-pain cycle. Option 2: Analgesics given too early can prolong labor. Options 3 and 4: These are not helpful or encouraging to the client; she obviously needs immediate attention of some kind.

NP: Assessment
CN: Psychosocial integrity
CNS: Coping and adaptation
CL: Application

69 A 24-year-old gravida 2 asks the nurse about the safety and effectiveness of a pudendal block. Which of these statements about a pudendal block would be most helpful to the client?

- ☐ 1. "A 6-inch needle is used to inject anesthetic into your vagina."
- ☐ 2. "A pudendal block often causes the mother's pulse to increase temporarily."
- ☐ 3. "A pudendal block can't be given until the baby's head is far down in the birth canal."
- ☐ 4. "There is usually little effect on the baby or on the course of labor."

CORRECT ANSWER: 4

A pudendal block contains a moderate dose of anesthetic, which has minimal effects on the fetus or on labor unless inadvertently injected intravenously. Option 1: The response is not worded sensitively; the client need not know the needle's exact length. Option 2: A pudendal block does not usually cause changes in maternal vital signs. Option 3: A transvaginal pudendal block is performed before the fetal head is far down in the birth canal.

NP: Implementation
CN: Physiological integrity
CNS: Pharmacological and parenteral therapies
CL: Comprehension

---

70 A first-time mother-to-be is in the labor room, her husband at her bedside. The client states that her contractions began 6 hours ago. Which of the following assessment findings would confirm that the client is in true labor?

- ☐ 1. Discomfort located chiefly in the abdomen
- ☐ 2. Constant intensity of contractions
- ☐ 3. Contractions occurring every 10 to 15 minutes and lasting 20 to 30 seconds
- ☐ 4. Cervix that is 100% effaced and 2 cm dilated

CORRECT ANSWER: 4

In true labor, the cervix becomes effaced and dilated. In false labor, contractions are located chiefly in the abdomen (Option 1), the intensity of contractions remains the same (Option 2), and the interval between contractions remains long (Option 3).

NP: Assessment
CN: Health promotion and maintenance
CNS: Growth and development through the life span
CL: Application

---

71 A client in labor is informed that she is going to receive epidural analgesia. She asks the nurse about disadvantages to this procedure. What is the nurse's best response?

- ☐ 1. "Fetal distress is a frequent problem."
- ☐ 2. "The incidence of operative delivery may be increased."
- ☐ 3. "The amount of blood loss is excessive."
- ☐ 4. "Only partial motor paralysis develops."

CORRECT ANSWER: 2

An epidural block takes 10 to 20 minutes to relieve pain and can result in maternal hypotension, decreased variability of the FHR, and increased incidence of operative delivery if the woman cannot bear down effectively. Option 1: Fetal distress is rare unless the mother experiences hypotension. Option 3: Blood loss is not excessive. Option 4: This is not a disadvantage; the mother is alert, responsive, and relaxed.

NP: Implementation
CN: Physiological integrity
CNS: Pharmacological and parenteral therapies
CL: Application

72 A 24-year-old client on the labor unit is being coached in the Lamaze method by her husband. On assessment, the nurse finds the client to be 5 cm dilated, 90% effaced, at +1 station with contractions coming every 2 to 3 minutes and lasting 35 to 40 seconds. The client has asked for pain relief. What is the nurse's best action?

☐ 1. Check maternal blood pressure and pulse and FHR in response to contractions.
☐ 2. Realize that it is too early to give pain medication, and encourage the husband to continue with the Lamaze coaching.
☐ 3. Arrange for a sonogram to determine fetal position.
☐ 4. Perform a vaginal examination to determine dilation, effacement, and station.

CORRECT ANSWER: 1
Before administering medication to a client in labor, the nurse must assess the client and fetus. Option 2: Pain medication can be given when the client is in active labor. Option 3: A sonogram is inappropriate for a client in labor. Option 4: The vaginal examination had just been performed and therefore is not necessary at this time.

NP: Assessment
CN: Health promotion and maintenance
CNS: Growth and development through the life span
CL: Application

---

73 A primigravida in labor for 13 hours clenches her fists, tightens her muscles, and screams during every contraction. Her reaction to labor seems exaggerated compared to the contraction pattern recording from the EFM. What is the nurse's best response?

☐ 1. Explain to the client that the EFM shows mild contractions, so she should just relax and let the contractions work.
☐ 2. Take over as her coach because her husband is not helping her properly.
☐ 3. Ignore her reactions, realizing that this is her first time in labor and her reactions will soon match the intensity of contractions shown on the EFM.
☐ 4. Palpate her abdomen to determine the intensity of labor contractions as they are taking place.

CORRECT ANSWER: 4
Internal and external fetal monitors are helpful in assessing the duration and frequency of contractions, but the external monitor does not accurately portray the intensity of the contraction. The labor room nurse must evaluate this by palpation. Options 1, 2, and 3 fail to recognize the need for palpation. Furthermore, Option 2 inappropriately suggests that the nurse take over the husband's role as coach.

NP: Assessment
CN: Health promotion and maintenance
CNS: Growth and development through the life span
CL: Analysis

---

74 A client is to have a cesarean section because of continuous vaginal bleeding and an abnormal FHR tracing. Which of the following would be the best preoperative medication for this client?

☐ 1. Meperidine (Demerol)
☐ 2. Oxytocin (Pitocin)
☐ 3. Promethazine (Phenergan)
☐ 4. Glycopyrrolate (Robinul)

CORRECT ANSWER: 4
Glycopyrrolate is a parasympatholytic that will decrease the risk of aspiration. Meperidine (Option 1) and promethazine (Option 3) can cause newborn CNS and respiratory depression. Oxytocin (Option 2) will precipitate labor.

NP: Implementation
CN: Physiological integrity
CNS: Pharmacological and parenteral therapies
CL: Analysis

75 A client is in the second trimester of her first pregnancy. Which of the following findings should the nurse bring to the attention of the obstetrician or nurse midwife?

☐ 1. Diagonal conjugate of 12.5 cm
☐ 2. Fundal height of 22 cm on August 20 (LMP = March 20)
☐ 3. Rubella titer (HAI) of 1:10.
☐ 4. No ballottement

CORRECT ANSWER: 4
Ballottement should be felt from the fourth to fifth month; no ballottement would suggest oligohydramnios and thus should be referred for further evaluation of fetal status. Options 1, 2, and 3 are normal findings.
NP: Assessment
CN: Health promotion and maintenance
CNS: Growth and development through the life span
CL: Analysis

---

76 A client in the active phase of labor has a reactive fetal monitor strip and has been encouraged to walk. When she returns to bed for a monitor check, she complains of a need to push. While performing a vaginal examination, the nurse accidentally ruptures the membranes, and as she withdraws her hand, the fetal cord comes out. What should the nurse do next?

☐ 1. Put the client in a knee-chest position.
☐ 2. Call the physician.
☐ 3. Push down on the uterine fundus.
☐ 4. Set up for fetal blood sampling to detect fetal acidosis.

CORRECT ANSWER: 1
The knee-chest position gets the weight of the baby off the cord to prevent disruption of blood flow. Options 2 and 4 are important, but they have a lower priority than getting the baby off the cord. Option 3 would increase danger by compromising cord blood flow.
NP: Application
CN: Physiological integrity
CNS: Physiological adaptation
CL: Analysis

---

77 A client with hypotonic labor dysfunction is receiving oxytocin augmentation. Her contractions become more frequent and intense. Dilation progresses to 8 cm, but the fetal head remains at station +1. The nurse notes a soft bulge just above the symphysis. Which of the following is the best nursing action?

☐ 1. Re-evaluate the fetal presentation.
☐ 2. Change the client's position.
☐ 3. Offer a narcotic analgesic.
☐ 4. Help the client urinate.

CORRECT ANSWER: 4
Assessment data indicate a full bladder that may impede fetal descent. Options 1, 2, and 3 are inappropriate because they do not address the assessment findings.
NP: Implementation
CN: Physiological integrity
CNS: Reduction of risk potential
CL: Analysis

78 A baby girl is delivered at 38 weeks' gestation. She weighs 5 lb, 2 oz and is having difficulty maintaining body temperature. Which nursing activity would best prevent cold stress in a term newborn?

☐ 1. Immediately after birth, dry the newborn thoroughly, place her in a radiant heater, and monitor her temperature for the next 2 hours.
☐ 2. Administer oxygen for the first 30 minutes of life.
☐ 3. Decrease integumentary stimulation after birth.
☐ 4. Maintain the environmental temperature at 30°C.

CORRECT ANSWER: 1

This helps prevent loss of body heat from evaporation, conduction, and convection. Options 2 and 3 would have no effect in preventing cold stress. Option 4 could still cause loss of body heat via conduction and convection.

NP: Implementation
CN: Physiological integrity
CNS: Physiological adaptation
CL: Application

---

79 In which of the following instances is it safe to continue an oxytocin (Pitocin) induction?

☐ 1. Contractions are painful to the mother.
☐ 2. Contractions last 100 seconds or more.
☐ 3. Contractions occur every 90 seconds.
☐ 4. The FHR is 100 beats/minute.

CORRECT ANSWER: 1

Maternal pain is not in itself an unsafe condition. Painful uterine contractions can be controlled with analgesia. Options 2 and 3: Contractions of this duration or frequency could cause fetal hypoxia. Option 4: This slowed FHR is a sign of fetal hypoxia.

NP: Implementation
CN: Physiological integrity
CNS: Pharmacological and parenteral therapies
CL: Comprehension

---

80 A gravida 2, para 1 with PIH is receiving magnesium sulfate I.V., 2 grams/hour via infusion pump. In assessing the client, the nurse notes a decrease in respirations from 16 to 12 breaths/minute and slightly pink-tinged urine (output is 25 ml/hour). The client still complains of feeling sleepy. The nurse's action should include which of the following?

☐ 1. Check the most recent serum level of magnesium sulfate, and notify the physician of the results.
☐ 2. Turn the client on her left side and take vital signs again.
☐ 3. Flush the client's indwelling urinary catheter with sterile normal saline solution to see if it is draining properly.
☐ 4. Instruct the client to turn, cough, and deep breathe every 30 minutes.

CORRECT ANSWER: 1

Urine that is scant (less than 30 ml/hour) and tinged with blood indicates potential renal damage and must be reported to the physician. Option 2 increases blood perfusion to the uterus. Option 3 is unnecessarily invasive and does not address the blood-tinged urine. Option 4 has nothing to do with the client's symptoms.

NP: Implementation
CN: Physiological integrity
CNS: Pharmacological and parenteral therapies
CL: Analysis

81 A client at term arrives in the labor room experiencing contractions every 4 minutes. While she is in active labor, the EFM registers a pattern indicating a variable deceleration. Which nursing intervention should be initiated first?

- ☐ 1. Monitor blood pressure every 5 minutes.
- ☐ 2. Change maternal position.
- ☐ 3. Increase I.V. fluid rate.
- ☐ 4. Prepare for an immediate cesarean section.

CORRECT ANSWER: 2

A variable deceleration usually indicates fetal cord compression. Changing the mother's position usually relieves the pressure on the cord, thereby increasing blood flow to the fetus. Option 1: Alterations in maternal blood pressure are not correlated with variable decelerations. Option 3: Increasing the I.V. fluids could increase placental perfusion but would not be the best first action. Option 4: An occasional or isolated variable deceleration is not an indication for an emergency cesarean delivery.

NP: Implementation
CN: Physiological integrity
CNS: Physiological adaptation
CL: Analysis

---

82 The community health center physician has confirmed that a 16-year-old client is at 16 weeks' gestation. The client confides to the nurse that she is afraid to tell her parents she is pregnant. Which of the following best explains the client's feelings?

- ☐ 1. The client lacks a stable relationship with her family.
- ☐ 2. The client fears rejection by her family because of her unplanned pregnancy.
- ☐ 3. The client's parents may force an abortion.
- ☐ 4. The client cannot rely on her family for emotional support.

CORRECT ANSWER: 2

The adolescent's perception of parental response causes fear of rejection. Parents' initial reactions to the news of their daughter's pregnancy are usually shock, anger, shame, guilt, and sorrow. However, in general, adaptation occurs as the pregnancy progresses, and the adolescent's mother usually becomes her key support system. Options 1 and 4: No data in this case study indicate abnormally unstable or nonsupportive family relationships. Option 3: The evidence given is insufficient to warrant such a conclusion at this point.

NP: Evaluation
CN: Psychosocial integrity
CNS: Coping and adaptation
CL: Application

83 The nurse should anticipate which psychological reactions during the second trimester of pregnancy?

☐ 1. Self-centeredness and concentration on the behavior and appearance of children
☐ 2. Extroversion and emotional lability
☐ 3. Ambivalence and uncertainty
☐ 4. Dismay over body image and readiness for the end of pregnancy

CORRECT ANSWER: 1
Women during the second trimester are somewhat narcissistic; at the same time, they commonly are fascinated by children. Option 2: Extroversion is a personality trait not specific to pregnancy; emotional lability may be present in every trimester. Option 3: This is characteristic of the first trimester. Option 4: This is characteristic of the third trimester.

NP: Assessment
CN: Health promotion and maintenance
CNS: Growth and development through the life span
CL: Application

---

84 As the newborn nursery nurse, you are responsible for the initial feeding of a newborn. You give a feeding of plain sterile water. The mother asks why this was given. What is your best response?

☐ 1. "Plain sterile water will cause less irritation to the respiratory tract if the baby accidentally breathes some in and is preferred until the baby's ability to feed is assessed."
☐ 2. "The doctor always orders this."
☐ 3. "Glucose water would give the baby too many calories."
☐ 4. "Formula and breast milk should be withheld for 12 hours after birth."

CORRECT ANSWER: 1
Plain sterile water is best for the initial feeding because it is less irritating to the respiratory tract if any is accidentally aspirated. Glucose water and formula, if aspirated, can cause an inflammatory response and pneumonia. Option 2: This peremptory response does not give any explanation to the client. Option 3: The caloric content of glucose water is not a threat to the newborn. Option 4: The issue is not how long to withhold feeding, but to assess in the safest way the baby's ability to feed.

NP: Implementation
CN: Health promotion and maintenance
CNS: Growth and development through the life span
CL: Analysis

---

85 A 7-lb, 4-oz baby boy is born by spontaneous vaginal delivery. During the initial assessment at 1 hour postpartum, the nurse notices lanugo, acrocyanosis, mongolian spots, and hemangiomas. Which of these is an abnormal finding in a newborn?

☐ 1. Lanugo
☐ 2. Acrocyanosis
☐ 3. Mongolian spots
☐ 4. Hemangiomas

CORRECT ANSWER: 4
Hemangiomas are vascular tumors considered deviations from the norm. Options 1, 2, and 3 are normal findings in a newborn.

NP: Assessment
CN: Health promotion and maintenance
CNS: Growth and development through the life span
CL: Application

86 If toxic levels of magnesium sulfate are reached, which of the following is the antidote of choice?

- ☐ 1. Terbutaline (Brethine)
- ☐ 2. Calcium gluconate (Kalcinate)
- ☐ 3. Hydralazine (Apresoline)
- ☐ 4. Dopamine (Intropin)

CORRECT ANSWER: 2

Calcium gluconate is the antidote for magnesium sulfate toxicity. Option 1: Terbutaline is a tocolytic used in the treatment of preterm labor. Option 3: Hydralazine is an antihypertensive used in the treatment of PIH. Option 4: Dopamine is an adrenergic agonist frequently used to treat hypotension.

NP: Implementation
CN: Physiological integrity
CNS: Pharmacological and parenteral therapies
CL: Comprehension

---

87 A baby weighing 1,500 g is born at 32 weeks' gestation. During an assessment at 12 hours of age, the nurse notices these signs and symptoms in the newborn: hyperactivity, persistent shrill cry, frequent yawning and sneezing, and jitteriness. These symptoms would indicate which of the following?

- ☐ 1. Sepsis
- ☐ 2. Hepatitis
- ☐ 3. Drug dependence
- ☐ 4. Hypoglycemia

CORRECT ANSWER: 3

These classic symptoms of a drug-dependent neonate usually appear within the first 24 hours of life. Options 1, 2, and 4 are not indicated by the given signs and symptoms.

NP: Assessment
CN: Physiological integrity
CNS: Physiological adaptation
CL: Analysis

---

88 A client is attempting a VBAC. Her contractions are 2 to 3 minutes apart, lasting from 75 to 100 seconds. Suddenly, the client complains of an intense abdominal pain, and the fetal monitor stops picking up contractions. The nurse recognizes that which of the following has occurred?

- ☐ 1. Abruptio placentae
- ☐ 2. Prolapsed cord
- ☐ 3. Partial placenta previa
- ☐ 4. Complete uterine rupture

CORRECT ANSWER: 4

The client would feel a sharp pain in the lower abdomen, and contractions would cease. FHR would also cease within a few minutes. Option 1: Uterine irritability would continue on the fetal monitor tracing with abruptio placentae. Option 2: Contractions would continue with a prolapsed cord, and there would be no pain from the prolapse itself. Option 3: There would be vaginal bleeding with a partial placenta previa but no pain outside of the expected pain of contractions.

NP: Assessment
CN: Physiological integrity
CNS: Physiological adaptation
CL: Application

89 Which of the following statements accurately describes the respiratory tract of newborns?

☐ 1. Newborns are mouth breathers.

☐ 2. Newborns have a low level of respiratory tract secretions.

☐ 3. Newborns have large tongues compared to the glottis and trachea.

☐ 4. Newborns have well-developed respiratory muscles.

CORRECT ANSWER: 3

Newborns have large tongues when compared to the glottis and trachea. Option 1: Newborns are nose breathers. Option 2: Newborns have an abundance of respiratory secretions. Option 4: Newborns have muscles that support respirations, but they are not well developed.

NP: Assessment

CN: Health promotion and maintenance

CNS: Growth and development through the life span

CL: Application

---

90 A client in active labor has received epidural anesthesia for pain. Nursing care for her during the epidural block should include which of the following?

☐ 1. Give the client 500 to 1,000 ml of lactated Ringer's solution intravenously 20 minutes after the block.

☐ 2. Position her flat on her back after the block to decrease leakage of spinal fluid.

☐ 3. Record the client's vital signs and the FHR every 1 to 2 minutes for the first 15 minutes after the block.

☐ 4. Avoid vaginal examinations to reduce exposing the epidural site to infection.

CORRECT ANSWER: 3

Maternal hypotension is a major complication of epidural anesthesia. This side effect can be minimized by elevating the right hip with pillows and by hydrating the mother before the procedure. The nurse needs to monitor vital signs and FHR every 1 to 2 minutes for at least 15 minutes after the block is completed. Option 1: Hydration should occur 20 minutes before the procedure, not 20 minutes after. Option 2: The right hip needs to be elevated to displace uterine pressure on the vena cava. Option 4: Vaginal examinations would not expose the site to infection.

NP: Implementation

CN: Physiological integrity

CNS: Reduction of risk potential

CL: Application

---

91 A client delivered her first child vaginally and her second child by cesarean section. She is now attempting a VBAC. As she labors, she freely admits to the nurse how frightened she feels. What is the nurse's best response?

☐ 1. "There is nothing to fear; someone will be with you all the time."

☐ 2. "I'll go get your husband. He will help you to feel less frightened."

☐ 3. "Did you say you are feeling frightened?"

☐ 4. "Don't worry, the doctor won't let anything happen to you."

CORRECT ANSWER: 3

This is an open-ended question that allows the client to explain why she is frightened. Option 1 patronizes the client. Options 2 and 4 stop the flow of communication.

NP: Implementation

CN: Psychosocial integrity

CNS: Coping and adaptation

CL: Application

92 A Type 1 diabetic is in labor. The physician prescribes 10 units of regular insulin I.V. in 1,000 ml of dextrose 5% in normal saline. You set up the insulin infusion on an infusion pump with a 10 drops/ml solution set. If you set the pump to deliver 100 ml/hour, how many units of insulin are you giving per hour?

☐ 1. 1
☐ 2. 1.5
☐ 3. 2
☐ 4. 5

CORRECT ANSWER: 1

$$\frac{\text{X units}}{\text{100 ml/hour}} = \frac{\text{10 units}}{\text{1,000 ml}}$$

$$X = \frac{\text{10 units}}{\text{1,000 ml}} \times \text{100 ml}$$

$$X = \text{1 unit}$$

NP: Planning
CN: Physiological integrity
CNS: Pharmacological and parenteral therapies
CL: Application

---

93 A baby boy is delivered with low forceps because of his mother's inability to push effectively during Stage II labor, secondary to epidural anesthesia. The baby is assessed by the nursing staff immediately after delivery and receives an Apgar score of 9 at 5 minutes after birth (-1 point for color). What does this Apgar score mean?

☐ 1. The baby is in a stable physiological state.
☐ 2. The baby may have a cardiovascular defect.
☐ 3. The baby may have an Rh incompatibility with its mother.
☐ 4. The baby may have a bleeding disorder that merits additional assessment.

CORRECT ANSWER: 1
An Apgar score of 9 is consistent with the interpretation of a healthy baby early in life. Option 2: Depending on the defect, symptoms would warrant a lower score. Option 3 and 4: No data in the case study support these conclusions.
NP: Assessment
CN: Health promotion and maintenance
CNS: Growth and development through the life span
CL: Application

---

94 At 6 cm cervical dilation, a client in labor tells the nurse that she would like to have an epidural. Which of the following nursing interventions should occur before an epidural is started?

☐ 1. Apply cardiac monitoring leads to the client's chest.
☐ 2. Ask the client to empty her bladder if she hasn't voided recently.
☐ 3. Assess the client's back for bony abnormalities or skin infection.
☐ 4. Prepare the client for insertion of a fetal scalp electrode.

CORRECT ANSWER: 2
The urge to void is diminished during an epidural block, and most women are unable to void. Emptying the bladder before administration of the epidural may prevent an unnecessary catheterization. Option 1: Close monitoring of blood pressure is necessary, but not of the cardiac rhythm. Option 3: It is the physician's responsibility to assess the potential epidural site and determine if its condition constitutes a contraindication. Option 4: External monitoring is usually adequate for fetal assessment.
NP: Planning
CN: Physiological integrity
CNS: Pharmacological and parenteral therapies
CL: Application

95 A postpartal client plans to breast-feed her first child, a full-term neonate. She asks the nurse, "How will I know if my baby is getting enough to eat?" The nurse tells her that she will know the baby is getting adequate nutrition if he:

- ☐ 1. wets six to eight diapers in 24 hours.
- ☐ 2. cries to be fed every 1 to 2 hours.
- ☐ 3. gains weight steadily.
- ☐ 4. burps after a feeding.

CORRECT ANSWER: 3

Signs that a neonate is getting adequate nutrition include a steady weight gain, 10 to 12 wet diapers every 24 hours, and contented behavior after a feeding. Options 1 and 2: Wetting only six to eight diapers in 24 hours and crying to be fed every 1 to 2 hours signal inadequate intake. Option 3: Burping after a feeding is not related to feeding adequacy.

NP: Implementation
CN: Health promotion and maintenance
CNS: Growth and development through the life span
CL: Comprehension

---

96 A 5-lb, 2-oz baby girl is delivered at 38 weeks' gestation by a mother with PIH of a month's duration. The baby is having difficulty maintaining a stable body temperature. Although she was delivered at term, the baby is being observed and cared for in the progressive nursery because of the physician's concerns about temperature instability. Which factor is most relevant to a term baby's inability to maintain a stable body temperature?

- ☐ 1. The baby's blood vessels are more internally located than those of an adult, so the baby responds less strongly to environmental temperatures.
- ☐ 2. The baby has a smaller ratio of body surface area to body mass.
- ☐ 3. The baby compensates for heat loss by shivering and therefore becomes acidotic.
- ☐ 4. The vasomotor center of a baby is relatively immature.

CORRECT ANSWER: 4

Because of the immaturity of the vasomotor center, the baby cannot shiver to compensate for heat loss. Option 1: Newborn temperature is highly subject to environmental temperature changes. Option 2: The newborn has a large surface area relative to body weight. Option 3: Shivering in the newborn is rare.

NP: Assessment
CN: Physiological integrity
CNS: Physiological adaptation
CL: Application

97 A client delivers a full-term infant by cesarean section, necessitated by cephalopelvic disproportion. The baby receives Apgar scores of 9 and 9. Immediately after delivery, a nurse assesses the mother. Which nursing diagnosis should be given priority?

- ☐ 1. Fluid volume deficit related to nothing-by-mouth status
- ☐ 2. Risk for fluid volume deficit related to potential hemorrhage
- ☐ 3. Pain related to incision
- ☐ 4. Impaired gas exchange related to general anesthesia and pain

CORRECT ANSWER: 4

Gas exchange is the primary concern during the immediate postoperative care of a client who has undergone a cesarean section. Options 1, 2, and 3 are important considerations, but they do not take top priority.

NP: Implementation
CN: Physiological integrity
CNS: Reduction of risk potential
CL: Analysis

---

98 The nurse palpates a newborn's palate with her index finger before feeding. This assessment is done in order to detect which of the following?

- ☐ 1. Sucking reflex
- ☐ 2. Opening in the palate
- ☐ 3. Epstein's pearls
- ☐ 4. Tooth buds

CORRECT ANSWER: 2

Palate deformities can cause aspiration during feeding, which may lead to such complications as pneumonia. Options 1, 3, and 4 are possible findings, but they are not priority assessments before initiating feeding.

NP: Assessment
CN: Health promotion and maintenance
CNS: Growth and development through the life span
CL: Comprehension

---

99 Which of the following is the priority assessment of a client receiving epidural anesthesia?

- ☐ 1. Maternal hypotension
- ☐ 2. Maternal tachycardia
- ☐ 3. Fetal tachycardia
- ☐ 4. Maternal diuresis

CORRECT ANSWER: 1

The most common complication of an epidural block is maternal hypotension. Option 2: This is not a direct result of epidural anesthesia, but it could occur as a compensatory mechanism if the client becomes hypotensive. Option 3: The fetus must be assessed for late decelerations, which could result from maternal hypotension. Option 4: Epidural anesthesia does not cause diuresis.

NP: Assessment
CN: Physiological integrity
CNS: Pharmacological and parenteral therapies
CL: Application

100 A primigravida client is admitted to the labor and delivery unit. She has attended three childbirth classes. On examination, the nurse finds that she is only 3 cm dilated. The physician decides to rupture her membranes artificially. As soon as the physician leaves the room, the client asks the nurse if she can have her epidural now so she won't feel any discomfort during labor. What is the nurse's best response?

☐ 1. "I'll call the anesthetist for you."
☐ 2. "If an epidural is given this early, it will most likely slow your labor."
☐ 3. "It's not time for this type of medication yet."
☐ 4. "It takes 15 to 20 minutes to take effect, so it's good to have it early."

CORRECT ANSWER: 2

Regional anesthesia slows labor if administered before the active phase. Most authorities do not recommend it before the mother is at least 5 cm dilated. Option 1: It is too early to give the anesthesia. Option 3: This gives the client no explanation. Option 4: Epidural anesthesia usually takes effect in 3 to 5 minutes.

NP: Implementation
CN: Health promotion and maintenance
CNS: Growth and development through the life span
CL: Analysis

---

101 A premature newborn weighs 4 lb. His mother asks the primary nurse which formula provides the best nutrition. The nurse has the choice of three calorie concentrations: 13, 20, or 24 calories/oz. Which of these formulas would be best for the newborn?

☐ 1. 13 calories/oz because it provides the most fluid
☐ 2. 20 calories/oz because it provides the best combination of fluid and calories
☐ 3. 24 calories/oz because it provides greater calories in less volume
☐ 4. None of these because the baby is too little to receive formula

CORRECT ANSWER: 3

The preterm infant's nutritional demands are best met by higher calorie, higher protein formulas, although not so high that they tax the ability of the immature kidneys to concentrate urine. Option 1: The caloric concentration is not adequate. Option 2: The caloric concentration is better, but still not adequate. Option 4: If the baby has a sufficient sucking reflex, he is large enough to receive formula.

NP: Planning
CN: Health promotion and maintenance
CNS: Growth and development through the life span
CL: Application

---

102 If a pregnant woman has a monilial infection at the time of vaginal delivery, what will the newborn most probably contract?

☐ 1. Retrolental fibroplasia
☐ 2. Vesicular skin lesions
☐ 3. Respiratory distress syndrome
☐ 4. Thrush

CORRECT ANSWER: 4

Monilia or *Candida albicans* causes thrush in the newborn delivered vaginally. Option 1: Retrolental fibroplasia, which commonly results in blindness, typically occurs in the preterm infant exposed to high oxygen levels. Option 2: Vesicular skin lesions appear with herpes. Option 3: Respiratory distress syndrome is caused by a lack of surfactant in the lungs.

NP: Assessment
CN: Physiological integrity
CNS: Reduction of risk potential
CL: Comprehension

103 A student nurse in the newborn nursery is assigned to a baby boy who has just been transferred to the nursery from the delivery room. She will begin to evaluate the newborn by assessing gestational age. Which two components comprise the gestational age rating tool?

☐ 1. Newborn reflexes and behavioral characteristics
☐ 2. Birthing history and the number of weeks from the date of the pregnant woman's last menstrual cycle
☐ 3. Apgar score and external physical characteristics
☐ 4. External physical characteristics and neuromuscular development

CORRECT ANSWER: 4
The external physical characteristics are objective clinical criteria not generally influenced by labor and birth and unlikely to change during the first 24 hours after birth. Neuromuscular examination facilitates assessment of functional or physiological maturation. Option 1: The nervous system is unstable, and neurological examination based on reflexes alone may not be reliable. Option 2: Gestational age "by dates" is only 75% to 85% accurate. The gestational age maturity rating tool is a more reliable system of evaluating the newborn. Option 3: Apgar score can be influenced by labor and birth.

NP: Assessment
CN: Health promotion and maintenance
CNS: Growth and development through the life span
CL: Application

---

104 Which of the following characterize the first period of reactivity in a newborn?

☐ 1. Awake and alert; period lasts 4 to 6 hours; newborn indicates readiness for feeding by rooting and sucking.
☐ 2. Awake and active; period lasts 30 minutes; newborn has a strong sucking reflex.
☐ 3. Activity diminished; heart rate and respirations decreased; no interest in sucking.
☐ 4. Stable vital signs; period lasts 2 to 4 hours; newborn will tolerate the first feeding well during this period.

CORRECT ANSWER: 2
These characteristics exemplify the first period of reactivity. During this time, bowel sounds are absent. Option 1: This typifies the second period of reactivity. Option 3: This behavior is characteristic of the sleep phase. Option 4: The first period of reactivity is much shorter than 2 to 4 hours.

NP: Assessment
CN: Health promotion and maintenance
CNS: Growth and development through the life span
CL: Comprehension

105 A client delivers a boy by spontaneous vaginal delivery. When assessing the client 2 days later, the nurse should expect to see which type of vaginal discharge?

☐ 1. Lochia rubra
☐ 2. Lochia serosa
☐ 3. Lochia alba
☐ 4. Non-lochia bleeding

Correct answer: 1
Postpartal uterine discharge is called lochia. Lochia rubra consists mostly of blood and decidual debris and occurs during the first 3 postpartal days. Option 2: Lochia serosa is pink or brown and begins after 3 or 4 days postpartum. It consists of old blood, serum, and leukocytes. Option 3: Lochia alba is yellow to white and occurs after 10 days postpartum. It consists of leukocytes, serum, and mucus. Option 4: Non-lochia bleeding, such as that from a cervical tear, is not a normal clinical finding.

NP: Assessment
CN: Health promotion and maintenance
CNS: Growth and development through the life span
CL: Application

---

106 Which of the following would be likely in a client who is 10 weeks pregnant if her cervix is dilated and she is having slight vaginal bleeding?

☐ 1. Complete abortion, because the membranes have ruptured
☐ 2. Habitual abortion, because this is the second lost pregnancy
☐ 3. Imminent abortion, because there is cervical dilation, bleeding, and cramping
☐ 4. Threatened abortion, because all the products of conception are expelled

Correct answer: 3
This is an accurate description of an imminent abortion. Option 1: A complete abortion would involve the loss of all the products of conception. Option 2: Habitual abortion applies to the loss of three consecutive pregnancies. Option 4: A threatened abortion involves unexplained bleeding and, possibly, cramping or backache, but no cervical dilation.

NP: Assessment
CN: Physiological integrity
CNS: Physiological adaptation
CL: Application

---

107 The nurse is performing postpartal teaching with a client as part of discharge planning. Which of the following statements about puerperal infection is important to discuss?

☐ 1. It can occur only during the lochia rubra phase.
☐ 2. It is common and will resolve spontaneously.
☐ 3. It can occur weeks after delivery; such symptoms as fever must be reported to the physician.
☐ 4. It includes mastitis.

Correct answer: 3
Puerperal infection can occur from immediately after delivery until the 28th postpartal day. Early symptoms are chills and fever; prompt treatment is important. Option 1: The infection can occur long after the lochia rubra phase has ended. Option 2: The condition is uncommon but potentially serious; it needs prompt treatment. Option 4: Puerperal infection refers only to infections of the genital tract.

NP: Planning
CN: Health promotion and maintenance
CNS: Growth and development through the life span
CL: Application

108 A client at 36 weeks' gestation has been on tocolytic agents to prevent preterm labor for the past month. She vaginally delivers a 6-lb, 2-oz girl, who is now in the NICU with respiratory distress and in need of supplemental oxygen via an oxygen hood. The mother is extremely concerned about her preterm baby and is crying in the postpartum recovery room. What statement by the nurse at this time would be most therapeutic?

☐ 1. "Your baby will be fine; her weight is appropriate for your length of pregnancy."
☐ 2. "I know how difficult this must be for you. I had an aunt whose baby died when she delivered early."
☐ 3. "You may be feeling helpless and overwhelmed now with these things you may not have expected."
☐ 4. "I'm sure you are glad to have the labor over since you had to take medication for so long to avoid labor."

CORRECT ANSWER: 3
This addresses the feelings that the client is probably experiencing, allows the client to verbalize more freely, and conveys acceptance of her feelings. Option 1: This gives false reassurance. Option 2: Such a statement about an aunt whose baby died is highly inappropriate. Option 4: This nonsupportive statement does not deal with the client's feelings.

NP: Implementation
CN: Psychosocial integrity
CNS: Coping and adaptation
CL: Application

---

109 A client is concerned about her figure returning after delivery. What teaching by the nurse can best assist the client in understanding and accepting appropriate post-delivery weight loss?

☐ 1. The abdominal muscles will return to their nonparous state at about 6 weeks after birth.
☐ 2. Weight loss and physiological stability can be attained by consuming about 1,000 calories a day.
☐ 3. Weight should be lost easily during the 6 weeks after delivery because of a consistently high basal metabolic rate.
☐ 4. A rigorous exercise program can play a predominant role in allowing a 30-lb weight loss in the first 6 weeks after birth.

CORRECT ANSWER: 1
This can be taught to the client postpartum. Option 2: A 1,000-calorie/day diet is severely restrictive and does not meet the basal metabolic needs of most adult women, let alone nursing mothers. Option 3: This is an inaccurate statement. Option 4: Vigorous exercise should not be attempted until after healing occurs. In any case, a 30-lb weight loss in 6 weeks is not safe.

NP: Implementation
CN: Health promotion and maintenance
CNS: Growth and development through the life span
CL: Application

110 A 25-year-old woman and her husband are at the obstetrician's office for a prenatal visit. The client, in the 32nd week of her third pregnancy, is complaining of urinary frequency and has a purulent vaginal discharge. She is diagnosed with gonorrhea. Which of the following is the best response by the nurse to the client's question, "How did I get this?"

☐ 1. "This is a sexually transmitted disease."
☐ 2. "Ask your husband where he got it."
☐ 3. "Where do you think you got it?"
☐ 4. "Have you had any partners other than your husband?"

CORRECT ANSWER: 1
This straightforward response provides the client with necessary information. The nurse can then assess further learning needs and offer the client support. The other options do not respond to the client's question. Further, Options 2 and 4 are judgmental.
NP: Implementation
CN: Psychosocial integrity
CNS: Coping and adaptation
CL: Analysis

---

111 A nurse assessing a newborn obtains these measurements: head circumference, 13 inches; chest circumference, 15 inches; abdominal circumference, 12 inches; and length, 20 inches. Which measurement deviates from the normal range?

☐ 1. Head
☐ 2. Chest
☐ 3. Abdomen
☐ 4. Length

CORRECT ANSWER: 2
The normal measurement for the chest is 12 to 13 inches. Options 1, 3, and 4 are normal measurements.
NP: Assessment
CN: Health promotion and maintenance
CNS: Prevention and early detection of disease
CL: Application

---

112 A client who vaginally delivered a boy 48 hours ago asks the nurse when she can resume sexual intercourse. What is the nurse's best response?

☐ 1. "When your vaginal discharge has stopped and your episiotomy is healed."
☐ 2. "Six weeks after delivery."
☐ 3. "After your scheduled postpartal check-up with your physician."
☐ 4. "Ask your doctor what he recommends."

CORRECT ANSWER: 1
To decrease the chance of infection and pain, intercourse should be postponed until the lochia stops and the episiotomy is healed. Option 2: Generally, healing is completed and the lochia ceases within 3 to 4 weeks. Options 3 and 4: There is no reason to wait until seeing the doctor, which may not happen until the routine checkup at 6 weeks postpartum. Anticipatory guidance is best; provide the client with an explanation and rationale for when intercourse can safely be resumed.
NP: Implementation
CN: Health promotion and maintenance
CNS: Prevention and early detection of disease
CL: Application

113 Two days after delivery, a client suddenly starts crying frequently for no apparent reason. The nurse should plan care based on which of the following?

☐ 1. Severe postpartum psychosis is frequent, and every client must be assessed for it.
☐ 2. The majority of women are depressed for a year or more after giving birth.
☐ 3. One outburst does not warrant any concern and need not be followed up on.
☐ 4. Transitory depression begins 2 days after birth, and the symptoms usually abate within the first week.

CORRECT ANSWER: 4
This is the typical pattern, although some women may take up to a year to fully resolve their feelings. Option 1: Severe psychosis occurs in fewer than 3% of women who have had normal deliveries. Option 2: The majority of postpartal women feel better emotionally after the first week. Option 3: Each woman's psychological and emotional health must be assessed following childbirth, especially when she shows signs of anxiety or tearfulness.

NP: Planning
CN: Psychosocial integrity
CNS: Coping and adaptation
CL: Application

---

114 One hour after a primigravida has given birth to a baby girl, the nurse is performing a physical assessment. When assessing fundal height, she would expect the fundus to be located at which level?

☐ 1. At the umbilicus
☐ 2. At the symphysis pubis
☐ 3. Midway between the umbilicus and the xiphoid process
☐ 4. Midway between the umbilicus and the symphysis pubis

CORRECT ANSWER: 4
The fundus should assume this position soon after delivery. The fundus rises to the level of the umbilicus a few hours later and stays there for a day. It then descends into the pelvis at a rate of about 1 fingerbreadth per day. Option 1: This is the height of the fundus at delivery. Option 2: The fundus will not reach this point until after the 10th day postpartum. Option 3: The fundus should not be this high.

NP: Assessment
CN: Health promotion and maintenance
CNS: Growth and development through the life span
CL: Comprehension

115 A gravida 3, para 2 client is admitted to the labor suite at 33 weeks' gestation. She is having contractions every 5 minutes, lasting 50 seconds. Membranes are intact; her cervix is not effaced but is 2 cm dilated. She is given ritodrine (Yutopar), a tocolytic used to interrupt preterm labor. Four hours after the ritodrine infusion is started, the client complains of feeling nervous and jittery. She expresses concern about these feelings. What is the nurse's best response?

☐ 1. "You seem bothered by this; I'll stop the I.V."
☐ 2. "You need this medication to stop the contractions; we must keep the I.V. infusing."
☐ 3. "This feeling of nervousness must be disturbing to you. Sometimes women get these kinds of feelings when they are on this medication."
☐ 4. "I'll call the doctor; this usually doesn't happen."

CORRECT ANSWER: 3

Common side effects of ritodrine are tremors, jitteriness, and nervousness. Preterm labor itself produces anxiety as well. The client needs psychosocial support and information given in an empathetic, caring manner. Option 1: The infusion should be continued, with close monitoring of vital signs to detect an increase in symptoms. Option 2: While accurate, this answer does not provide emotional support. Option 4: These side effects are common.

NP: Implementation
CN: Physiological integrity
CNS: Pharmacological and parenteral therapies
CL: Application

---

116 The nurse is assessing a baby 4 hours old. Which of the following would be a cause of concern?

☐ 1. Anterior fontanel is 2 cm wide, head is molded, and sutures are overriding.
☐ 2. Hands and feet are cyanotic, abdomen is rounded, and the infant has not voided or passed meconium.
☐ 3. Color is dusky, axillary temperature is 97° F, and the baby is spitting up excessive amounts of mucus.
☐ 4. Respirations are irregular and abdominal in character, and the baby has intermittent tremors of the extremities when crying.

CORRECT ANSWER: 3

Skin color is expected to be pink tinged or ruddy, saliva should be scant, and the normal axillary temperature ranges from 97.7° F to 98.6° F. Option 1: The anterior fontanel measures 2 to 3 cm wide by 3 to 4 cm long. Overriding sutures and molding, when present, may persist for a few days after birth. Option 2: Acrocyanosis may be present for the first 2 to 6 hours after birth. The infant would be expected to pass meconium and void within the first 24 hours. Option 4: Neonatal tremors are common in the full-term neonate; however, they must be evaluated to differentiate them from a convulsion or evidence of such problems as hypoglycemia or hypocalcemia.

NP: Assessment
CN: Health promotion and maintenance
CNS: Growth and development through the life span
CL: Application

117 A 35-year-old client is in the 8th month of her first pregnancy. The physician is conducting a biophysical profile. In a 20-minute period during the nonstress test (NST), the baby experiences four periods of spontaneous fetal movement associated with an increase in the FHR of 20 beats/minute over the baseline rate. What would be the results of the NST?

☐ 1. Nonreactive
☐ 2. Reactive
☐ 3. Equivocal
☐ 4. Negative

CORRECT ANSWER: 2
The spontaneous fetal movement and increased FHR indicate a reactive NST. Options 1, 3, and 4 are incorrect.
NP: Evaluation
CN: Health promotion and maintenance
CNS: Growth and development through the life span
CL: Analysis

---

118 During discharge planning, a postpartal client asks her primary nurse what exercises she could begin in order to prevent "female problems with urination" in the future. What should the nurse encourage the client to do?

☐ 1. Begin modified situps at least three times daily.
☐ 2. Hold urine inside to improve bladder tone.
☐ 3. Contract the pelvis before lifting heavy objects.
☐ 4. Contract and relax the perineum frequently.

CORRECT ANSWER: 4
Perineal tightening (Kegel) exercises tighten the pubococcygeal muscle, which improves support to the pelvic organs and helps regain sphincter tone. Option 1: It is too soon for her to begin situps, and they will not help strengthen the perineal muscles. Option 2: Voluntarily retaining urine can promote infection; it is not recommended. Option 3: This will not help improve perineal muscle tone.
NP: Implementation
CN: Health promotion and maintenance
CNS: Growth and development through the life span
CL: Application

---

119 During discharge teaching, a postpartal client tells her nurse that she feels very irritable, depressed, and tearful. What would be the nurse's best response?

☐ 1. "These feelings are normal and usually decrease after the first week or two."
☐ 2. "You will feel better when you get home and have a good night's sleep."
☐ 3. "You should tell your physician if you still feel depressed at your 6-week check-up."
☐ 4. "You will feel better if you invite family and friends over for coffee."

CORRECT ANSWER: 1
Postpartum blues occur in 50% of primigravidas and usually are short-lived. Option 2: It is unlikely that the new mother will get a good night's sleep; even if she did, this alone would not resolve her feelings. Option 3: The client should be contacted shortly after discharge, via telephone or a home health visit. Persistent symptoms may indicate a serious depression. The client should not have to wait 6 weeks for further evaluation. Option 4: Although the support of friends and family is helpful, the client should not feel the burden of having to entertain them.
NP: Implementation
CN: Health promotion and maintenance
CNS: Growth and development through the life span
CL: Application

120 A 17-year-old primigravida at 36 weeks' gestation has been brought to the emergency department complaining of lower abdominal cramps. The nurse asks for a clean-catch urine sample for urinalysis and a urine culture. What is the purpose of urinalysis?

☐ 1. A positive nitrite value indicates the presence of bacteria.
☐ 2. A urinalysis is necessary before doing a culture.
☐ 3. High urine pH can cause preterm labor.
☐ 4. There is no significance.

CORRECT ANSWER: 1

Irritability from a bladder infection can initiate preterm labor and lead to uncomfortable contractions. Urinalysis results are obtained quickly and can suggest enough evidence of a bladder infection to warrant immediate treatment. By contrast, a urine culture takes 24 to 36 hours for a preliminary report and up to 72 hours for a final report. Option 2: While a urine culture is necessary to determine the causative agent of the infection, the urinalysis allows treatment to begin before the culture results are obtained. Option 3: High urine pH is not linked to preterm labor. Option 4: Untreated infections can jeopardize the health of the mother and the fetus.

NP: Assessment
CN: Physiological integrity
CNS: Reduction of risk potential
CL: Comprehension

---

121 A client asks the nurse when she might expect the stretch marks on her abdomen to disappear. What is the nurse's best response?

☐ 1. "They'll be gone in a few weeks."
☐ 2. "They will soon begin to fade to a lighter colors — silver or white."
☐ 3. "They are never going to go away; you'll just have to live with them."
☐ 4. "If you keep rubbing them with cocoa butter cream, they'll disappear faster."

CORRECT ANSWER: 2

Stretch marks, also called striae, will gradually fade to silver or white streaks. Option 1: Stretch marks do not disappear completely. Option 3: This is a very nonsupportive answer. Option 4: Cocoa butter will not help the stretch marks disappear.

NP: Implementation
CN: Health promotion and maintenance
CNS: Growth and development through the life span
CL: Application

122 In performing a vaginal exam on a client in labor, the nurse discovers that the fetus's larger, diamond-shaped fontanel is toward the anterior portion of the pelvis. What does this finding tell the nurse?

☐ 1. The client can expect a brief and intense labor, with potential for lacerations.
☐ 2. The client is at risk for uterine rupture and needs constant monitoring.
☐ 3. The client may need interventions to ease back labor and change the fetal position.
☐ 4. The client needs to be told that the fetus will have to be delivered with forceps.

CORRECT ANSWER: 3
The fetal position is occiput posterior, which commonly produces intense back pain during labor. Most of the time, the fetus rotates during labor from occiput posterior to occiput anterior position. Positioning the mother on all fours can facilitate this rotation. Option 1: Occiput posterior would most likely result in prolonged labor. Option 2: This position does not create a particular risk of uterine rupture. Option 4: The fetus would have to be delivered with forceps only if it does not rotate spontaneously.

NP: Planning
CN: Health promotion and maintenance
CNS: Growth and development through the life span
CL: Analysis

---

123 A 15-year-old primigravida at 30 weeks' gestation is admitted to the hospital. She lives at home with her mother and attends a local prenatal program. She is underweight, has poor nutritional habits, and smokes a half pack of cigarettes per day. Her chief complaints on arrival are heavy cramps and a severe backache. At the initial vaginal exam, the client's cervix is soft, 70% effaced, and 1 cm dilated. According to standard premature labor protocol, the nurse would initiate which of the following actions?

☐ 1. Send the client home to maintain bed rest.
☐ 2. Allow the client to ambulate to determine whether cramping will continue or stop.
☐ 3. Admit the client, maintain her in a lateral position in bed, and hydrate her with a 500-ml I.V. solution.
☐ 4. Perform a vaginal exam every 15 minutes to determine cervical change.

CORRECT ANSWER: 3
Bed rest in a lateral position relieves cervical pressure and may reduce the frequency and intensity of contractions. Hydration is important because it can decrease the release of antidiuretic hormone and oxytocin from the posterior pituitary gland. Option 1: The client should not be sent home because she may not comply with the physician's orders for bed rest; besides, she needs hydration and ongoing assessment to rule out labor. Option 2: Ambulation should be avoided because it puts pressure on the cervix, increasing the risk of further dilation. Option 4: Frequent cervical manipulation may increase the intensity of contractions.

NP: Implementation
CN: Health promotion and maintenance
CNS: Growth and development through the life span
CL: Application

124 A woman anticipating a cesarean delivery asks the nurse about advantages of a lower transverse uterine incision. What is the nurse's best response?

☐ 1. "Having this incision may allow a woman to deliver vaginally in a subsequent pregnancy."
☐ 2. "It generally heals more quickly than other types of uterine incisions."
☐ 3. "The bladder is not in the way as much as with a classic incision."
☐ 4. "This incision can be performed quickly, as in emergency situations."

CORRECT ANSWER: 1
Lower transverse uterine incisions are the least likely to rupture during subsequent labors. Option 2: They do not heal more quickly than other incisions. Option 3: The bladder must be dissected away from the uterus when a lower transverse uterine incision is performed. Option 4: Because of the need to dissect the bladder away from the uterus, the lower transverse uterine incision cannot be performed as quickly as the classic incision.

NP: Implementation
CN: Health promotion and maintenance
CNS: Growth and development through the life span
CL: Application

---

125 While the nurse is providing discharge instructions, a postpartal cesarean section client asks what her chances are of having a VBAC with her next pregnancy. What is the nurse's best response?

☐ 1. "Women who plan to have epidural anesthesia for labor should not consider a VBAC."
☐ 2. "Women who had cesareans for cephalopelvic disproportion are discouraged from having a VBAC."
☐ 3. "Women who had postoperative complications should not consider a VBAC."
☐ 4. "Women who had a low transverse uterine incision are candidates for a VBAC."

CORRECT ANSWER: 4
Low transverse uterine incisions are less likely to rupture in subsequent labors than other types of incisions. Option 1: Although some practitioners prefer to offer less medication, epidural anesthesia is not contraindicated for a VBAC. Options 2 and 3: These are not automatic disqualifications for a VBAC.

NP: Implementation
CN: Health promotion and maintenance
CNS: Growth and development through the life span
CL: Application

---

126 A client in labor with her second baby is 5 cm dilated. The physician has diagnosed hypotonic labor dysfunction and plans an oxytocin augmentation. What is the nurse's priority intervention?

☐ 1. Maintain placental circulation.
☐ 2. Promote maternal comfort.
☐ 3. Observe fluid balance.
☐ 4. Evaluate cervical dilation and effacement.

CORRECT ANSWER: 1
Intense contractions that can result from oxytocin stimulation may reduce placental blood flow. Options 2, 3, and 4 are all important, but maintaining oxygen flow to the fetus through placental circulation is the highest priority.

NP: Planning
CN: Physiological integrity
CNS: Growth and development through the life span
CL: Analysis

127 After a client has a cesarean section, the nurse can best prevent hemorrhagic shock by doing which of the following?

☐ 1. Check blood pressure, pulse, and respirations every 15 minutes.

☐ 2. Assess and maintain a firm uterine contraction.

☐ 3. Limit narcotic analgesia.

☐ 4. Check for bleeding on the dressing.

CORRECT ANSWER: 2

Uterine atony is the most likely cause of postpartum hemorrhage, whether the birth was cesarean or vaginal. This complication is best prevented by checking the fundus for firmness to evaluate whether the uterine muscle is compressing the open vessels at the placental site. Option 1: This would detect shock but not prevent it. Option 3: This would have no effect on the occurrence of shock and would likely cause the client needless distress. Option 4: This is an appropriate action, but incisional disruption is not as likely a cause of hemorrhage as uterine atony.

NP: Implementation
CN: Physiological integrity
CNS: Reduction of risk potential
CL: Application

---

128 A 7-lb, 6-oz male is born with a unilateral cleft lip and complete cleft palate. What should be the nurse's primary concern during the newborn's initial feeding?

☐ 1. Observe the newborn's respiratory rate and color.

☐ 2. Assess the mother's comfort level during the feeding.

☐ 3. Measure the amount of formula the newborn takes.

☐ 4. Assess the parents' interaction with the newborn.

CORRECT ANSWER: 1

Infants with cleft lip and palate commonly have sucking and swallowing problems. Aspiration is a danger, so respiratory assessment would be the nurse's initial priority. Options 2, 3, and 4 are important, but none would take precedence over respiratory assessment.

NP: Assessment
CN: Physiological integrity
CNS: Reduction of risk potential
CL: Analysis

Child Nursing

1 A 2-year-old male is admitted through the emergency room with a suspected diagnosis of Hirschsprung's disease (aganglionic megacolon). The child's mother asks about treatment of the disease. The nurse's response should be based on which of the following?

☐ 1. He will have a permanent colostomy; as he matures, he can learn the required care.
☐ 2. He will have a temporary colostomy; "pull-through" surgery will be done in the future.
☐ 3. He will require many reconstructive colostomy surgeries over a lifetime.
☐ 4. He will require chemotherapy and radiation to treat his disease.

CORRECT ANSWER: 2
Repair of aganglionic megacolon requires dissection of the aganglionic segment and anastomosis with the unaffected intestine. It is usually done in a two-stage operation. The first surgery creates a colostomy to evacuate the bowel of stool and rest the distended portion of the bowel. The second surgery, done several months later, involves colostomy closure and a rectal "pull-through." Option 1: The colostomy is not permanent. Option 3: Only a two-stage operation is required. Option 4: Chemotherapy and radiation are never required for this condition; it is not cancer.

NP: Planning
CN: Physiological integrity
CNS: Physiological adaptation
CL: Application

---

2 An obese 14-year-old girl states that she wants to lose weight. Besides her dietary intake and physical activity, which of the following would be the most important to assess?

☐ 1. Her metabolic rate
☐ 2. Who prepares the meals
☐ 3. How food is used in her home
☐ 4. Her educational interests

CORRECT ANSWER: 3
Food habits and eating behaviors are largely related to cultural patterns and family preferences. Options 1 and 4: Although these data might be useful in motivation, they do not add to the dietary history. Option 2: It would be better to assess the complete nutritional environment, including such factors as the school cafeteria.

NP: Assessment
CN: Health promotion and maintenance
CNS: Prevention and early detection of disease
CL: Application

3 A 15-year-old girl with bulimia complains to the nurse that all the other girls on the ward are nerds. What is the best action for the nurse to take?

- ☐ 1. Explain how the client's attitude affects the other girls.
- ☐ 2. Sit her down and ask her why she doesn't like the other girls.
- ☐ 3. Include boys and girls in her age group when planning activities.
- ☐ 4. Help her select activities that include the nurse and other teenagers.

Correct answer: 4

Having her participate in activity selection gives her some control over her life while in the hospital. Clients with an eating disorder have difficulty with issues of control, so an opportunity to allow them to participate in the therapeutic program helps. Options 1 and 2 may easily provoke a defensive response by the client. Option 3 is not as therapeutic as allowing her to help choose activities.

NP: Planning
CN: Psychosocial integrity
CNS: Coping and adaptation
CL: Application

---

4 A newborn is assessed by the nursery nurse for congenital dislocated hip. Which of the following is the most reliable assessment for this condition?

- ☐ 1. Trendelenburg's test
- ☐ 2. Curvature of the lower spine
- ☐ 3. Macewen's sign
- ☐ 4. Ortolani's click

Correct answer: 4

Ortolani's click is a reliable sign of hip dislocation in the newborn. Option 1: Trendelenburg's test is used to assess the valves of the leg veins. Option 2: Curvature of the spine is more directly associated with scoliosis. Option 3: Macewen's sign is a neurologic assessment for hydrocephalus.

NP: Assessment
CN: Health promotion and maintenance
CNS: Growth and development through the life span
CL: Application

---

5 A 3-year-old male comes to the ambulatory care clinic with his father for a routine visit. He has a runny nose and a cough. The father tells the nurse of a family history of asthma and eczema. What findings should the nurse assess for when auscultating the child's chest?

- ☐ 1. A prolonged inspiratory phase of the respiratory cycle
- ☐ 2. A shortened expiratory phase of the respiratory cycle
- ☐ 3. Marked inspiratory stridor
- ☐ 4. Rhonchi, especially on expiration, which is prolonged

Correct answer: 4

By history and symptomatology, the nurse would suspect that this child might have signs of bronchial asthma, which is manifested by bronchospasm and prolonged expiration. Options 1 and 2: A child with this history and symptomatology would have a shortened inspiratory phase and prolonged expirations. Option 3: Inspiratory stridor is more likely found in croup.

NP: Assessment
CN: Health promotion and maintenance
CNS: Prevention and early detection of disease
CL: Application

6 The mother of a 3-year-old boy calls the hospital to report that her child has ingested a few acetaminophen (Tylenol) tablets. She has a poison kit with syrup of ipecac and activated charcoal at home. The family lives approximately 1 hour's drive from the hospital. What should the nurse instruct the mother to do?

☐ 1. Administer 15 ml of syrup of ipecac orally, followed by 200 to 300 ml of fluid to induce vomiting; then bring the child to the hospital.
☐ 2. Administer 30 ml of syrup of ipecac orally, followed by 8 to 16 ounces of fluid to induce vomiting; don't leave for the hospital until the child has vomited a large amount.
☐ 3. Administer 10 g of activated charcoal, followed by 4 to 8 ounces of milk to absorb the toxin; then bring the child to the hospital.
☐ 4. Rush the child to the hospital immediately, where professional treatment will be started as soon as he arrives.

CORRECT ANSWER: 1

This is the correct dosage of ipecac and amount of fluid recommended to induce vomiting and eliminate the poison from a 3-year-old. Option 2: The amounts of ipecac and fluids are excessive for a preschooler. Also, 90% of children vomit within 30 minutes of the appropriate dose of ipecac; waiting for vomiting to occur would delay stomach gavage and administration of the antidote. Option 3: Activated charcoal should not be given with milk products, and then only when evacuation of stomach contents is unsafe. Option 4: Acetaminophen is rapidly absorbed from the GI tract, with peak levels at 1 to 2 hours after ingestion. Failure to evacuate the stomach contents increases the risk of organ damage and death.

NP: Implementation
CN: Physiological integrity
CNS: Pharmacological and parenteral therapies
CL: Analysis

---

7 A 2-year-old male is admitted for possible bacterial meningitis. Which of the following nursing actions should the nurse take first?

☐ 1. Read the client's history and physical examination report.
☐ 2. Assess the client's neurologic status.
☐ 3. Interview the client's mother and father.
☐ 4. Administer oxygen at 3 liters/minute by nasal cannula.

CORRECT ANSWER: 2

Acute meningitis can be a pediatric emergency. A diagnosis based on accurate assessments is a priority for correct treatment. A baseline neurologic assessment is needed for later comparisons. Options 1 and 3: These are not a priority in comparison to neurologic status. Option 4: No orders nor data exist to warrant this action.

NP: Assessment
CN: Physiological integrity
CNS: Reduction of risk potential
CL: Application

---

8 A 10-year-old girl with sickle cell anemia has been admitted for vaso-occlusive crisis. Which of the following would be the best activity for the client?

☐ 1. Bowling
☐ 2. Stringing beads on yarn
☐ 3. Swimming
☐ 4. Painting

CORRECT ANSWER: 4

During a vaso-occlusive crisis, the child needs to minimize oxygen consumption. Painting is the only quiet and age-appropriate activity. Options 1 and 3 are too strenuous for a child in vaso-occlusive crisis. Option 2 is not an appropriate activity for a 10-year-old.

NP: Planning
CN: Physiological integrity
CNS: Reduction of risk potential
CL: Application

9 A 10-year-old male with sickle cell anemia has been an active fifth grader with good grades. When reviewing a plan of care, the nurse would expect to see which of the following prescribed in order to rebuild hemolyzed red blood cells (RBCs)?

- ☐ 1. Regular doses of folic acid
- ☐ 2. Prophylactic antibiotics to prevent cell damage
- ☐ 3. Daily iron-fortified vitamins
- ☐ 4. High doses of vitamin C

CORRECT ANSWER: 1

Folic acid helps rebuild RBCs without causing excessive levels of iron. Options 2 and 4: Neither antibiotics nor vitamin C will rebuild hemolyzed RBCs. Option 3: Iron-fortified vitamins can cause too high a level of iron.

NP: Implementation
CN: Physiological integrity
CNS: Pharmacological and parenteral therapies
CL: Application

---

10 A 6-year-old child is immunosuppressed from human immunodeficiency virus (HIV) infection. The nurse should emphasize that the parents not allow their child to come in contact with which of the following?

- ☐ 1. A school-age child who has scoliosis
- ☐ 2. A 16-year-old who has just received a tetanus booster
- ☐ 3. An infant who has just received an oral polio vaccine
- ☐ 4. A toddler who has eczema

CORRECT ANSWER: 3

The polio virus can be shed from the GI tract after administration of the oral vaccine. An immunosuppressed child should avoid contact with the virus, which is weakened but live. Options 1 and 4: Scoliosis and eczema are not contagious. Option 2: Tetanus vaccine is not live.

NP: Implementation
CN: Safe, effective care environment
CNS: Safety and infection control
CL: Analysis

---

11 A child with thalassemia major (Cooley anemia) is to receive a blood transfusion. Which of the following administration techniques represents safe nursing procedure?

- ☐ 1. Transfuse blood rapidly to complete the procedure as soon as possible.
- ☐ 2. Discontinue the transfusion and remove the I.V. needle if allergic symptoms develop.
- ☐ 3. Slow the drip rate if allergic symptoms develop.
- ☐ 4. Discontinue the transfusion but maintain the I.V. line if allergic symptoms develop.

CORRECT ANSWER: 4

If allergic symptoms develop, the transfusion should be discontinued, but the I.V. line should be maintained for administration of medications and fluids to counteract the allergic response. Option 1: Blood is transfused slowly for the first 15 minutes. Option 2: The I.V. line should be maintained for emergency treatment of allergic response. Option 3: The transfusion must be discontinued if allergic symptoms develop.

NP: Implementation
CN: Physiological integrity
CNS: Pharmacological and parenteral therapies
CL: Analysis

12 Which of the following would be a priority nursing diagnosis for a child with iron-deficiency anemia?

- ☐ 1. Activity intolerance related to reduced oxygen-carrying capacity of blood
- ☐ 2. Activity intolerance related to iron-deficiency anemia
- ☐ 3. Altered tissue perfusion (cardiopulmonary) related to hypervolemia
- ☐ 4. Altered tissue perfusion (peripheral) related to skin pallor

CORRECT ANSWER: 1

Reduced oxygen-carrying capacity of the blood in anemia decreases the energy available for normal activity. Option 2: Iron-deficiency anemia is a medical diagnosis; it is inappropriate in a nursing diagnosis statement. Option 3: Iron-deficiency anemia does not result in hypervolemia, which is an increase in blood volume. Option 4: Skin pallor is a sign of altered tissue perfusion and, therefore, a defining characteristic, not an etiology.

NP: Assessment
CN: Physiological integrity
CNS: Basic care and comfort
CL: Analysis

---

13 Which of the following would be most important to include when teaching home management of a child with hemophilia?

- ☐ 1. Toothbrushes should be held under warm water before use.
- ☐ 2. Aspirin should be used for mild joint pain and inflammation.
- ☐ 3. Bleeding extremities should be held in a dependent position to encourage stasis and clot formation.
- ☐ 4. Wall-to-wall carpeting should not be used anywhere in the home.

CORRECT ANSWER: 1

Softening the toothbrush under warm water decreases the risk of bleeding gums. Option 2: Aspirin is contraindicated because it interferes with platelet function. Option 3: Bleeding extremities should be kept elevated. Option 4: The home should have wall-to-wall carpeting to cushion falls.

NP: Implementation
CN: Physiological integrity
CNS: Reduction of risk potential
CL: Analysis

---

14 A child with iron-deficiency anemia is being treated with iron supplements. The client's mother brings the child to the clinic 3 months after iron supplements have been prescribed. The child's hematocrit level is about the same as it was 3 months ago. What information should the nurse first elicit from the mother?

- ☐ 1. A dietary history
- ☐ 2. A description of the child's stools
- ☐ 3. Whether the child has been exposed to sickle cell disease
- ☐ 4. Whether the child is pale and more tired than usual

CORRECT ANSWER: 2

The nurse must first determine if the child is receiving the iron supplements; stools that are green or black indicate that the child has been taking supplements. Option 1: A dietary history does not offer objective evidence that the child has received the iron supplements. Option 3: Sickle cell disease is a genetic trait, not a contagious disease. Option 4: Because the physical effects of anemia are insidious, parents may not view their child as ill or in need of treatment.

NP: Evaluation
CN: Physiological integrity
CNS: Physiological adaptation
CL: Analysis

15 An 18-month-old female comes in for a well-baby checkup. Her mother reports that she drinks five 8-oz bottles of whole milk a day. Which of the following should the nurse tell the mother to include in the child's diet to improve iron intake?

- ☐ 1. Peanut butter, green vegetables, and raisins
- ☐ 2. Cheese, yogurt, and fresh fish
- ☐ 3. Yellow vegetables, citrus fruits, and white bread
- ☐ 4. Berries, turkey, and cheese

CORRECT ANSWER: 1

Legumes, green vegetables, and dried fruits are high sources of iron. Options 2, 3, and 4 have a lower iron content.

NP: Implementation
CN: Health promotion and maintenance
CNS: Prevention and early detection of disease
CL: Application

---

16 A 10-year-old male with sickle cell anemia continues to wet the bed at night. He feels frustrated about this and is too embarrassed to sleep over at a friend's house. Which of the following responses by the nurse is most appropriate?

- ☐ 1. "We can try a bladder training program."
- ☐ 2. "Force fluids during the day and restrict fluids after 7:00 p.m."
- ☐ 3. "Decrease fluid intake during the day and take no liquids before bedtime."
- ☐ 4. "Perhaps your friends could sleep over at your house instead."

CORRECT ANSWER: 1

About half of all children with sickle cell anemia have problems with enuresis because the kidney is damaged and can no longer concentrate urine. Bladder training programs may improve the situation. Options 2 and 3: Restricting fluids in someone with sickle cell anemia can lead to a vaso-occlusive crisis. Option 4: This does not show understanding of the child's feelings.

NP: Planning
CN: Psychosocial integrity
CNS: Coping and adaptation
CL: Application

---

17 An 18-month-old's mother complains that the child seems tired and fussy even though she naps twice a day and sleeps through the night. The nurse notes that the child is pale and clinging to her mother during the health history and assessment. Which of the following findings should lead the nurse to suspect iron-deficiency anemia?

- ☐ 1. She drinks 40 to 48 oz of pasteurized cow's milk daily.
- ☐ 2. She weighed 8 lb, 9 oz when she was born.
- ☐ 3. She is often constipated, and her stool is very dark.
- ☐ 4. She is in the 50th percentile for height and the 60th percentile for weight.

CORRECT ANSWER: 1

A dietary history typically reveals abnormally high milk intake (over 32 oz of cow's milk daily). Option 2: Preterm infants are at greater risk for iron-deficiency anemia than babies born at full weight. Option 3: Constipation and dark stool may be associated with iron supplements, which are used to treat iron-deficiency anemia. Option 4: From 30% to 56% of children with iron-deficiency anemia are below the 10th percentile for weight when diagnosed.

NP: Assessment
CN: Health promotion and maintenance
CNS: Prevention and early detection of disease
CL: Analysis

18 A 4-year-old boy with acute lymphocytic leukemia has been receiving vincristine (Oncovin). Which of the following signs would be most important to the nurse in evaluating the side effects of vincristine therapy?

☐ 1. Diarrhea
☐ 2. Hematuria
☐ 3. Moon face and fluid retention
☐ 4. Weakness and constipation

CORRECT ANSWER: 4

Vincristine is a plant alkaloid. Neurotoxicity, a possible side effect of vincristine therapy, may be manifested as weakness and constipation. Option 1: Peristalsis is reduced, not increased, with vincristine; therefore, diarrhea is unlikely. Option 2: Hematuria is a side effect of cyclophosphamide (Cytoxan). Option 3: Moon face and fluid retention are side effects of prednisone (Sterapred).

NP: Assessment
CN: Physiological integrity
CNS: Pharmacological and parenteral therapies
CL: Application

---

19 A 4-year-old girl is admitted to the hospital to rule out leukemia. Which of the following would be the best room assignment?

☐ 1. With a 4-year-old girl who has rheumatoid arthritis
☐ 2. With a 5-year-old boy who is having a tonsillectomy
☐ 3. With a 4-year-old girl who has leukemia
☐ 4. Alone in a private room

CORRECT ANSWER: 4

Avoiding exposure to infection requires a private room. Options 1, 2, and 3: Cross-infection could occur from being with any of these children.

NP: Implementation
CN: Safe, effective care environment
CNS: Safety and infection control
CL: Application

---

20 A 2-year-old girl is being discharged from the hospital after treatment for croup. Her father asks, "What should we do if she gets croup again?" What is the best nursing response?

☐ 1. "You don't have to worry. She now has immunity to croup and will not get it again."
☐ 2. "Come to the emergency room immediately when she starts coughing."
☐ 3. "If she gets another cold, watch for croup. Keep a cool-mist humidifier running in her room, and give her lots of clear liquids."
☐ 4. "You could put her crib in the bathroom and let her sleep with the hot shower running to make steam."

CORRECT ANSWER: 3

A child can get croup again, particularly during an upper respiratory infection. The symptoms of croup may be relieved or lessened through adequate hydration and increased humidity. Option 1: An attack of croup does not confer immunity. Option 2: This may cause unnecessary parental anxiety and dependency on the health care provider; it does not teach how to control croup. Option 4: This is unsafe; a child should never be left alone in the bathroom with hot water running.

NP: Planning
CN: Physiological integrity
CNS: Reduction of risk potential
CL: Application

21 A newborn infant with a tracheoesophageal fistula (TEF) is to undergo a repair. Postoperatively, which of the following nursing measures should be implemented first?

☐ 1. Place the client in a prone position, with the head slightly elevated and turned to either side.
☐ 2. Place the client in a side-lying position, with the neck hyperextended to maintain an airway.
☐ 3. Give the first oral feeding with sterile water 24 hours after surgery.
☐ 4. Change the client's position every 2 hours from the back to either side, keeping the head slightly elevated.

CORRECT ANSWER: 4

The head is elevated to facilitate drainage of secretions. The position is changed frequently to maintain skin integrity and to prevent pneumonia. Option 1: The prone position compresses the abdomen and may cause gastric reflux. Option 2: Hyperextension of the neck puts pressure on the suture line of the esophagus. Option 3: Oral feedings are not started until 2 to 10 days after surgery.

NP: Implementation
CN: Physiological integrity
CNS: Reduction of risk potential
CL: Application

---

22 A 2-year-old client returns from surgery after a bowel resection as a result of Hirschsprung's disease. A temporary colostomy is in place. Which immediate postoperative nursing intervention for the client would have priority?

☐ 1. Change the surgical dressing.
☐ 2. Suction the nasopharynx frequently to remove secretions.
☐ 3. Irrigate the colostomy with 100 ml of normal saline solution.
☐ 4. Auscultate lung sounds.

CORRECT ANSWER: 4

The immediate nursing intervention after surgery would be to assess pulmonary function. Option 1: The surgical dressing should not require changing right away. Option 2: Suctioning should be performed only if the client cannot maintain a patent airway. Option 3: Colostomy irrigation is not warranted.

NP: Implementation
CN: Physiological integrity
CNS: Reduction of risk potential
CL: Application

---

23 A 2-week-old client returned 6 hours ago from surgery to correct pyloric stenosis. Which postoperative nursing management would be most important?

☐ 1. Feed small amounts frequently, assess the amount of emesis, and encourage parental involvement in care.
☐ 2. Give the infant nothing by mouth until the wound heals, and encourage parental involvement.
☐ 3. Monitor intake and output, and encourage parental involvement in care.
☐ 4. Monitor hydration status, and encourage parental involvement.

CORRECT ANSWER: 1

Small, frequent feedings are resumed 4 to 6 hours after surgery; the amount of and interval between feedings should gradually increase. Occasional emesis is common after surgery, and nurses need to let parents know about this. Parental involvement is a must, both preoperatively and postoperatively, to promote bonding and decrease feelings of guilt. Option 2: There is no reason to restrict oral feeding. Options 3 and 4: Assessing and developing feeding tolerance are of primary importance.

NP: Implementation
CN: Physiological integrity
CNS: Reduction of risk potential
CL: Application

24 A 1-month-old client is admitted to the hospital after 2 days of diarrhea and vomiting. The client is lethargic and has a weak pulse. Which action should be initiated first?

- ☐ 1. Obtain the health history.
- ☐ 2. Obtain a fuller history of the present illness.
- ☐ 3. Question the mother about formula preparation.
- ☐ 4. Initiate I.V. rehydration.

CORRECT ANSWER: 4

With moderate to severe diarrhea, the first aim is to restore vascular volume as rapidly as possible to prevent or treat shock. Options 1, 2, and 3 are important but do not take top priority.

NP: Planning
CN: Physiological integrity
CNS: Reduction of risk potential
CL: Analysis

---

25 A 2-month-old client with diarrhea and vomiting has been receiving I.V. fluids for the past 24 hours. The specific gravity of the client's urine is 1.012. What should the nurse do next?

- ☐ 1. Check the client's blood pressure.
- ☐ 2. Check the specific gravity again as soon as possible.
- ☐ 3. Notify the physician.
- ☐ 4. Continue the ordered I.V. flow rate.

CORRECT ANSWER: 4

The client's urine specific gravity is within normal limits, indicating that the baby is being adequately hydrated. Options 1, 2, and 3 are not necessary.

NP: Implementation
CN: Physiological integrity
CNS: Reduction of risk potential
CL: Analysis

---

26 A 4-year-old male is brought to the ambulatory care clinic for well-child care. His height (37 inches) and weight (29 lb) are below the 5th percentile for his age and sex. What should the nurse do first in evaluating his growth?

- ☐ 1. Compare his growth trends with those of his parents and siblings.
- ☐ 2. Elicit more history to assess the presence of metabolic disease.
- ☐ 3. Gather additional data by assessing baseline vital signs.
- ☐ 4. Initiate radiographic assessment to determine bone age.

CORRECT ANSWER: 1

A child who falls above or below the standard in both height and weight may not be abnormal but may reflect a genetically large or small frame. Comparing a child's growth trends with those of parents and siblings is essential in evaluating adequate growth. Options 2 and 4 may be appropriate in evaluating short stature, but they would not be the initial step. Option 3 might assist in the assessment of an underlying metabolic cause of short stature, but taking vital signs is not directly related to the initial evaluation of growth trends.

NP: Evaluation
CN: Health promotion and maintenance
CNS: Growth and development through the life span
CL: Analysis

27 A 15-month-old male is brought to the ambulatory care clinic for well-child care by his mother. He is crying and pulling at his left ear, which appears erythematous. Which of the following actions should the nurse take first?

☐ 1. Ask the mother to leave the room, because her anxiety is increasing the child's distress.
☐ 2. Examine the ear with the child supine, because this aids in visualizing the tympanic membrane.
☐ 3. Examine the affected ear last in order to minimize distress early in the exam.
☐ 4. Examine the left ear first in order to assess what may be physically wrong with the child.

CORRECT ANSWER: 3

The suggested sequence of a well-child exam may change considerably when the child is in pain. It is then preferable to examine the affected area last in order to minimize distress early in the exam and to focus on normal, healthy body parts. Option 1: Parental presence is almost always conducive to a child's cooperation and sense of security. Option 2: Examination of the ear in an upright position is preferable, especially in a crying child; it is less frightening for the child and decreases the bulging of the tympanic membrane from crying. Option 4: The painful body part should be examined last.

NP: Implementation
CN: Health promotion and maintenance
CNS: Prevention and early detection of disease
CL: Application

---

28 A healthy 6-year-old boy has never been immunized. His mother brings him to the clinic today to "get his shots for school." Which of the following immunizations should the client receive today?

☐ 1. MMR (measles, mumps, rubella)
☐ 2. DPT (diphtheria, tetanus, pertussis) and OPV (oral polio vaccine)
☐ 3. Hib (Haemophilus influenza type b)
☐ 4. DPT, OPV, and MMR

CORRECT ANSWER: 4

A child over 15 months and under 7 years with no previous immunizations should receive DPT, OPV, and MMR at the first visit. Options 1 and 2: These immunization plans would be incomplete. Option 3: The Hib vaccine is not given to children over 5 years old.

NP: Planning
CN: Health promotion and maintenance
CNS: Prevention and early detection of disease
CL: Application

---

29 A 2-year-old male is brought to the ambulatory care clinic by his father for a routine well-child visit. He has a runny nose and a cough. The nurse examines his musculoskeletal system. Which physical finding would indicate further investigation?

☐ 1. A broad-based gait
☐ 2. Asymmetric or unilateral bowleg
☐ 3. Knock-knee
☐ 4. Lordosis of the lower spine

CORRECT ANSWER: 2

Asymmetry of body parts is generally a clue to a problem. Unilateral bowleg that is present past the age of 2 may represent a pathologic condition. Options 1 and 4: A broad-based gait and lordosis are normal findings in a toddler. Option 3: Knock-knee is normally present in most children 2 to 7 years.

NP: Assessment
CN: Health promotion and maintenance
CNS: Prevention and early detection of disease
CL: Comprehension

30 Which of the following is the most significant finding in a history related to congenital hip dislocation?

☐ 1. The mother's activity during the third trimester
☐ 2. Breech presentation at birth
☐ 3. The client's serum calcium level at birth
☐ 4. An Apgar score of 4 at 1 minute and 6 at 5 minutes

CORRECT ANSWER: 2
Breech presentation is a factor frequently associated with congenital dislocated hip. Options 1, 3, and 4 have no bearing on hip dislocation.
NP: Assessment
CN: Health promotion and maintenance
CNS: Growth and development through the life span
CL: Application

---

31 Immediately after a 1-year-old client returns from a cardiac catheterization, the nurse notes that the pulse distal to the catheter insertion site is weaker. The nurse should take which of the following actions?

☐ 1. Remove the pressure bandage from the insertion site.
☐ 2. Perform passive exercises on the affected extremity.
☐ 3. Notify the physician of the assessment.
☐ 4. Record the data on the nursing notes.

CORRECT ANSWER: 4
The pulse distal to the insertion site may be weaker for a few hours but should gradually increase in strength. Option 1: The pressure dressing should not be removed because of the risk of hemorrhage. Option 2: Such exercises would not be performed after a cardiac catheterization. Option 3: The physician does not need to be notified at this time.
NP: Implementation
CN: Physiological integrity
CNS: Reduction of risk potential
CL: Analysis

---

32 A 12-month-old female client is at the clinic for a well-baby checkup. During the oral examination, the nurse discovers that the teeth are full of caries and that the client still uses a bottle. What is the nurse's most appropriate intervention?

☐ 1. Ask the client's mother about her knowledge of dental caries and bottle weaning.
☐ 2. Tell the client's mother that dental caries are caused by laying the baby down to sleep with a bottle full of milk.
☐ 3. Ask the client's mother about the client's bedtime routine.
☐ 4. Tell the client's mother to take the baby off the bottle and to see a dentist right away.

CORRECT ANSWER: 3
This open-ended question allows the nurse to gather information without attaching blame. Option 1: Asking the mother about her knowledge is likely to put her on the defensive. Option 2: This response is quick to assign blame. Option 4: The tone of this response is inappropriately peremptory.
NP: Implementation
CN: Health promotion and maintenance
CNS: Prevention and early detection of disease
CL: Application

33 A male client was born with a complete cleft palate and unilateral cleft lip. The client is now 2½ months old and has just returned to the unit from the recovery room after cleft lip repair. The recovery room nurse reports that his vital signs have been stable and he now is awake and active. What should be the unit nurse's initial intervention?

☐ 1. Take the client's vital signs.
☐ 2. Position the client on his abdomen.
☐ 3. Restrain the client's elbows.
☐ 4. Administer pain medication to decrease the client's activity.

Correct answer: 3

Because the baby is awake and active, the suture area must be protected. Option 1: Although vital signs are important, the recovery room nurse reported that they were stable; therefore, the restraints are more important at this time. Option 2: The client should not be positioned on his abdomen, as this can cause trauma to the suture line. Option 4: Pain medication may be required soon, but vital signs should be reassessed before it is administered.

NP: Implementation
CN: Physiological integrity
CNS: Reduction of risk potential
CL: Application

---

34 A 5-month-old female is brought to the pediatric clinic by her mother. The child has had recurrent middle-ear infections since she was 3 months old. Which of the following areas is most important to assess at today's visit?

☐ 1. How well the client eats
☐ 2. The client's weight gain since her last visit
☐ 3. Whether the client received all of her prescribed antibiotic at the time of the last infection
☐ 4. The client's temperature

Correct answer: 3

If the client is not receiving her full course of antibiotic therapy, her ear infections will recur; permanent hearing loss or systemic infection may result. Parents may not understand this and may discontinue treatment when the infant seems better. Options 1, 2, and 4 are important aspects to assess, but none is as critical as ensuring full compliance with antibiotic therapy.

NP: Assessment
CN: Physiological integrity
CNS: Pharmacological and parenteral therapies
CL: Analysis

---

35 A 3-year-old male child's mother calls the hospital emergency department, sobbing that he has swallowed some acetaminophen (Tylenol). In assessing the situation, the nurse's first priority is to learn which of the following?

☐ 1. How the child was able to gain access to the acetaminophen
☐ 2. Whether the child is complaining of right upper quadrant abdominal tenderness
☐ 3. Whether the child looks jaundiced
☐ 4. The number and strength of the acetaminophen tablets ingested

Correct answer: 4

Initial assessment requires finding out how much acetaminophen the child has ingested to determine whether the amount is toxic for his age and weight. Option 1: Safety measures should be taught after the emergency is resolved. Option 2: Right upper quadrant tenderness indicates liver toxicity, which would occur 1 or more days after ingesting a toxic amount of acetaminophen. Option 3: Jaundice would be a late sign of liver toxicity.

NP: Assessment
CN: Physiological integrity
CNS: Reduction of risk potential
CL: Analysis

36 Which of the following is the most desirable position for a newborn with a congenital dislocated hip?

- ☐ 1. Semi-Fowler's with both legs flexed
- ☐ 2. Legs adducted with head elevated
- ☐ 3. Swaddled in a baby carrier
- ☐ 4. Prone position with hips abducted

CORRECT ANSWER: 4

Abduction places the femoral head into the acetabulum for correct alignment. Options 1 and 2 do not help correct the problem. Option 3 would worsen the dislocation.

NP: Planning
CN: Physiological integrity
CNS: Reduction of risk potential
CL: Application

---

37 A 12-year-old boy with cystic fibrosis (CF) is tested for duodenal enzyme activity. Measurements reveal that he is deficient in trypsin. To replace the absent pancreatic enzyme, pancrelipase (Pancrease) is prescribed. The nurse should teach the client and parents that pancrelipase should be taken under what conditions?

- ☐ 1. On an empty stomach
- ☐ 2. Between meals
- ☐ 3. With meals and snacks
- ☐ 4. At bedtime

CORRECT ANSWER: 3

Trypsin is absent in over 80% of clients with CF. Pancreatic enzyme replacement is given with all meals and snacks to help digest food. Pancrelipase is enteric-coated to delay release of the enzyme and to prevent its destruction in the acid environment of the stomach. Capsules may be swallowed whole or broken apart and sprinkled on cold or room-temperature food. Options 1, 2, and 4: The enzyme should be given with food to aid in digestion.

NP: Implementation
CN: Physiological integrity
CNS: Pharmacological and parenteral therapies
CL: Comprehension

---

38 A 1-year-old male child is diagnosed with a congenital cardiac defect after cardiac catheterization. His parents have expressed concern about activities at home. Which is the best response by the nurse when teaching these parents?

- ☐ 1. "You will have to establish strict discipline so that he learns what he can't do."
- ☐ 2. "Allow him to play and be active as long as he doesn't get fatigued."
- ☐ 3. "He will only be able to play by himself."
- ☐ 4. "Discipline and limit-setting need to be relaxed to reduce his stress and crying."

CORRECT ANSWER: 2

Parents should promote normality within the limits of the child's condition. Options 1 and 4: The child needs to have appropriate limits and discipline. Being too strict with the child or overindulging him makes it hard for him to learn acceptable behavior. Option 3: Children of this age are beginning to explore their world and need to be exposed to activities with other children.

NP: Implementation
CN: Physiological integrity
CNS: Reduction of risk potential
CL: Application

39 A 7-month-old boy still has a congenitally displaced hip despite having been in a Frejka splint for 10 weeks. He is placed in a spica cast in a position of external rotation. Which of the following is most important to emphasize in teaching his parents how to care for him at home?

☐ 1. Avoid having plastic touch the edges of the cast.
☐ 2. Powder his perineal area with a medicated powder after each diaper change.
☐ 3. Check his circulation in both feet every hour.
☐ 4. Rock and cuddle him often.

CORRECT ANSWER: 4

Appropriate stimulation is needed to meet developmental needs. Holding, rocking, and cuddling help meet these needs by making the client feel cared for and secure. Option 1: The edges of the cast should be petaled to protect his skin from rough edges; the perineal area should be lined with plastic to protect the cast from urine and feces. Option 2: The use of powder should be discouraged, as it tends to cake under the cast. Option 3: This is appropriate for the first 24 hours he is in the cast; daily checks are recommended thereafter.

NP: Implementation
CN: Health promotion and maintenance
CNS: Growth and development through the life span
CL: Application

---

40 A 3-year-old boy is having the third and final surgery to repair a severe hypospadias. He returns from surgery with an I.V. of D_5W at 40 ml/hour, an indwelling urinary catheter to straight drainage, diet as tolerated, and pain medication as needed. Which of the following actions would be best for the nurse to take in order to prevent separation of the incision?

☐ 1. Place him in semi-Fowler's position.
☐ 2. Elevate the scrotal sac on a folded sheepskin.
☐ 3. Use restraints as needed to keep him from touching the area.
☐ 4. Clean the area every 2 hours with diluted hydrogen peroxide.

CORRECT ANSWER: 2

Elevation of the affected area on a Bellevue bridge or similar structure helps avert separation of the suture line by preventing dependent edema. Option 1: This will increase the swelling. Option 3: Staying with a 3-year-old client would be more appropriate than restraining him. Option 4: This would have no effect on incision separation.

NP: Implementation
CN: Physiological integrity
CNS: Reduction of risk potential
CL: Application

41 After a computed tomography (CT) scan, a lumbar puncture for spinal fluid collection is performed on a 2-year-old with bacterial meningitis. The lumbar puncture should not be performed if increased intracranial pressure (ICP) is reported in the CT scan in order to prevent which complication?

- ☐ 1. Herniating the brain stem
- ☐ 2. Spreading the organisms in the spinal fluid
- ☐ 3. Traumatizing the child with an additional test
- ☐ 4. Removing glucose from the already glucose-depleted spinal fluid

CORRECT ANSWER: 1

Removal of spinal fluid in the presence of increased ICP can cause downward displacement of the brain and damage tissue. Options 2 and 4: Lumbar puncture will not cause these conditions. Option 3: The procedure may be traumatic, but it is necessary for safe treatment and management of the child's condition.

NP: Planning
CN: Physiological integrity
CNS: Reduction of risk potential
CL: Analysis

---

42 A 3-year-old girl is brought to the emergency department by her father, who found her playing with an empty bottle of acetaminophen. The child said she had swallowed "a lot of the pills to help her feel better." Her father thinks the bottle was about two-thirds full of acetaminophen tablets for children. The nurse explains that she must try to empty the child's stomach of the drug by inserting a nasogastric (NG) tube. Which of the following measuring techniques would best ensure the correct tube length?

- ☐ 1. Measure from the tip of the nose to the earlobe, and from there to the end of the xiphoid process.
- ☐ 2. Measure from the tip of the earlobe to the end of the xiphoid process, and multiply by 2.
- ☐ 3. Measure from the tip of the nose to the umbilicus.
- ☐ 4. Measure from the tip of the nose to the umbilicus, and multiply by 2.

CORRECT ANSWER: 1

Correct measurements for insertion of an NG tube would be from the tip of the nose to the earlobe to the end of the xiphoid. Options 2, 3, and 4 would result in too long a tube.

NP: Assessment
CN: Physiological integrity
CNS: Physiological adaptation
CL: Comprehension

43 A 6-year-old girl has been hospitalized with rheumatic fever for 4 weeks. Her symptoms have gradually subsided, and she is now ready for discharge. Which of the following plans for her health care is most important for her future well-being?

☐ 1. Arrange for her to return to school as soon as possible to promote psychosocial development.

☐ 2. Encourage her to engage in unrestricted physical activity to regain physical strength.

☐ 3. Arrange for the administration of prophylactic antibiotics to prevent a recurrence of rheumatic fever.

☐ 4. Maintain seizure precautions, as central nervous system (CNS) involvement may persist for several months.

CORRECT ANSWER: 3

Children who have had rheumatic fever are more susceptible to contract it again. Prophylactic antibiotics are typically maintained for at least 5 years. Option 1: Psychosocial development can be promoted even before return to school is appropriate. Option 2: Physical activity should be limited until cardiac status is normal. Option 4: Choreic movements are not permanent and are not seizures.

NP: Planning
CN: Health promotion and maintenance
CNS: Growth and development through the life span
CL: Application

---

44 A female infant with acute bronchiolitis is on the pediatric unit, on nothing-by-mouth (NPO) status and receiving I.V. fluids. The mother asks, "Why can't she drink?" Which statement by the nurse best explains the reason for eliminating feedings at this time?

☐ 1. "She doesn't need as many calories now."

☐ 2. "There is a strong possibility of fluid overload."

☐ 3. "Feeding her now would be too much of an effort for her."

☐ 4. "Her digestive system has slowed down because of the infection."

CORRECT ANSWER: 3

Oral feedings during the acute phase of this illness will increase hypoxemia. The effort expended in feeding may result in tachypnea, weakness, and fatigue. Intravenous feedings are preferred during the acute phase. Option 1: During the acute phase, the client's caloric need will actually increase because of accelerated basal metabolism. Option 2: Although the nurse must continuously monitor hydration status to provide adequate hydration and prevent pulmonary edema, this is not the primary reason why the child is on NPO status at this time. Option 4: Increased peristalsis and acute diarrhea are commonly associated with infections outside the alimentary canal. The nurse would not expect peristalsis to decrease.

NP: Implementation
CN: Physiological integrity
CNS: Reduction of risk potential
CL: Application

45 The clothes of a 17-year-old male ignite while he is lighting the barbecue grill at a family picnic. His sister is a nurse. Which of the following actions should she take first?

☐ 1. Move her brother away from the barbecue grill.
☐ 2. Remove her brother's clothing.
☐ 3. Use the garden hose to put out the flames.
☐ 4. Call the fire department.

CORRECT ANSWER: 3
In emergency burn care, the priority is to stop the burning. Option 1: The client should not be moved because flames may intensify. Option 2: Once the fire is extinguished, the client's clothes will be removed, to prevent further injury. Option 4: Emergency medical personnel should be summoned after the flames are out.

NP: Implementation
CN: Safe, effective care environment
CNS: Safety and infection control
CL: Application

---

46 A client has third-degree burns of the hands, face, and chest. Which of the following nursing diagnoses would have priority?

☐ 1. Ineffective airway clearance related to edema
☐ 2. Body image disturbance related to physical appearance
☐ 3. Altered urinary elimination related to fluid loss
☐ 4. Infection related to epidermal disruption

CORRECT ANSWER: 1
When a client is admitted to the hospital with burns, the primary focus is on assessing and managing an effective airway. Options 2, 3, and 4 are integral parts of burn management but are not the first priority.

NP: Planning
CN: Physiological integrity
CNS: Physiological adaptation
CL: Analysis

---

47 A 13-year-old with structural scoliosis has had Harrington rods inserted. Which of the following would be the best postoperative position for the client?

☐ 1. Flat in bed
☐ 2. In a side-lying position
☐ 3. In semi-Fowler's position
☐ 4. In high Fowler's position

CORRECT ANSWER: 1
After placement of Harrington rods, the client must remain flat in bed. The gatch of a manual bed should be taped, and electric beds should be unplugged, to prevent the head or foot of the bed from being raised. Options 2, 3, and 4 would be detrimental to the success of the surgery because they would not maintain the spine in a straight position.

NP: Implementation
CN: Physiological integrity
CNS: Reduction of risk potential
CL: Application

48 The stool culture for a child with gastroenteritis is positive for rotavirus. Which of the following would the nurse expect to find during an assessment?

☐ 1. Ear tugging, ear drainage, and cervical lymph node enlargement
☐ 2. Positioning, eye movement, and crying
☐ 3. Strange food requests and additional use of salt
☐ 4. Altered respirations and abnormal breath sounds

CORRECT ANSWER: 4
Infants with gastroenteritis caused by rotavirus commonly have an accompanying respiratory condition. Option 1: These are signs and symptoms of otitis media, which is not as common with rotavirus as upper respiratory infections. Option 2: Neurologic complications are not common with rotavirus. Option 3: These nutritional assessments are not of particular concern.

NP: Assessment
CN: Physiological integrity
CNS: Physiological adaptation
CL: Analysis

---

49 A 13-year-old girl who has been diagnosed with structural scoliosis by her school nurse is fitted with a Milwaukee brace. How long should the nurse teach her that it must be worn?

☐ 1. 8 hours per day
☐ 2. 12 hours per day
☐ 3. 23 hours per day
☐ 4. 24 hours per day

CORRECT ANSWER: 3
The brace may be removed only 1 hour per day for bathing and hygiene. Options 1 and 2: These wearing times are too short to provide the necessary correction. Option 4: This does not allow for bathing or for skin integrity checks.

NP: Implementation
CN: Physiological integrity
CNS: Reduction of risk potential
CL: Knowledge

---

50 A 1-year-old child has been scheduled for cardiac catheterization. Which of the following would best prepare the child for the procedure?

☐ 1. Show the catheter insertion site on an anatomically correct doll the evening before the procedure.
☐ 2. Explain the procedure in very simple terms just before giving the preoperative medication.
☐ 3. Explain the procedure to the parents, who should provide support during stressful events.
☐ 4. Provide comfort and security when giving the preoperative medication.

CORRECT ANSWER: 4
Infants particularly need comfort to feel secure because they lack the cognitive skills to understand intrusive procedures. Options 1 and 2 would be appropriate for an older child. Option 3 assumes that the parents would provide support, which not all parents are able to do.

NP: Implementation
CN: Psychosocial integrity
CNS: Coping and adaptation
CL: Application

51 At a routine well-child assessment, a 2-year-old male manifests a runny nose and a cough. On examining the client's heart, the nurse records the findings listed below. Which one may be a sign of an abnormality?

☐ 1. A systolic, vibratory, high-pitched murmur that changes with the client's position

☐ 2. An arrhythmia that does not change when the client holds his breath

☐ 3. The point of maximal cardiac impulse apparent to visual inspection of the fifth intercostal space

☐ 4. The S_1 heart sound heard best at the apex of the client's heart

CORRECT ANSWER: 2

An abnormal arrhythmia can be differentiated from a sinus arrhythmia, which is commonly heard in children during inspiration and expiration, by listening to heart sounds as the child holds his breath. Option 1 describes a functional, nonorganic murmur common in children. Options 3 and 4 are normal findings.

NP: Assessment
CN: Health promotion and maintenance
CNS: Prevention and early detection of disease
CL: Application

---

52 A 12-year-old white male with CF presents with increased shortness of breath, increased cough and sputum production, fatigue, and weight loss. He is having trouble taking care of himself without exhaustion. Which approach by the nurse is most appropriate when setting goals?

☐ 1. Let the client set his own goals so that he will accomplish them.

☐ 2. Agree to follow what the physician says to do, regardless of what the client wants.

☐ 3. Tell the client what you would like him to accomplish so that he is aware of what is expected from him.

☐ 4. Agree on mutual goals to increase the client's sense of control in this situation.

CORRECT ANSWER: 4

Teens with a long-term fatal illness need as great a sense of control as possible. Option 1: Letting the client set goals completely on his own is not realistic, as he cannot fully comprehend all the medical aspects of his condition. Option 2: A holistic view of the client is of primary concern to the nurse; the physician is not the locus of control. Option 3: The nurse is not the primary locus of control either.

NP: Planning
CN: Psychosocial integrity
CNS: Coping and adaptation
CL: Application

---

53 A 1-year-old child has been diagnosed with postductal coarctation of the aorta and is admitted to the acute care unit for treatment of the heart defect. When performing an assessment, the nurse finds that the lower extremities are cool. Which finding should the nurse anticipate as the assessment continues?

☐ 1. Generalized irritability

☐ 2. Bilateral dilated pupils

☐ 3. Low blood pressure in the legs

☐ 4. Bilateral pedal edema

CORRECT ANSWER: 3

Postductal coarctation of the aorta causes diminished peripheral pulses, hypotension, and resulting cool temperature in the lower extremities. Options 1 and 2 are not related to postductal coarctation of the aorta. Option 4 is not related to diminished perfusion of the lower extremities.

NP: Assessment
CN: Physiological integrity
CNS: Physiological adaptation
CL: Application

54 Which of the following should the nurse teach the parents in helping to prevent rheumatic fever in their child?

☐ 1. Avoid exposing the child to streptococcal organisms.
☐ 2. Insist that a sore throat in the child be treated with antibiotics.
☐ 3. Learn the signs and symptoms of rheumatic fever.
☐ 4. Seek diagnosis and comply with treatment of recognizable streptococcal symptoms.

CORRECT ANSWER: 4

Prevention or treatment of group A streptococcal infection prevents rheumatic fever. Option 1 is not realistic; it is usually impossible to know when one is being exposed. Option 2 would be an inappropriate use of antibiotics; many sore throats are viral and would not respond to antibiotic treatment. Option 3 does nothing to prevent the occurrence of rheumatic fever.

NP: Implementation
CN: Health promotion and maintenance
CNS: Prevention and early detection of disease
CL: Comprehension

---

55 A 6-year-old female was treated 6 weeks ago for strep throat. She returns to the clinic with another sore throat and fever, and she now has a rash and complains of joint pain. She is admitted to the hospital with a tentative diagnosis of rheumatic fever. Which of the following strategies will best help prevent permanent damage?

☐ 1. Promote early ambulation to reduce joint stiffness and pain.
☐ 2. Maintain bed rest to reduce cardiac workload.
☐ 3. Limit visitors and maintain a quiet room to minimize CNS stimulation.
☐ 4. Avoid salicylates to avoid risk of Reye's syndrome.

CORRECT ANSWER: 2

The prognosis for rheumatic fever depends on the extent of myocardial involvement. Activity must be limited until cardiac status is normal. Option 1: There are no permanent aftereffects of joint involvement. Option 3: There are no permanent aftereffects of chorea. Option 4: Salicylates are prescribed for the pain and fever accompanying rheumatic fever, which is associated with antibodies to streptococcal bacteria. Reye's syndrome is associated with the use of salicylates for viral infections.

NP: Planning
CN: Physiological integrity
CNS: Reduction of risk potential
CL: Application

---

56 Which statement by a 15-year-old female client with CF should the nurse explore further?

☐ 1. "School is so boring this year."
☐ 2. "Sometimes I wonder if I am normal."
☐ 3. "I think I would like to be an astronaut more than anything."
☐ 4. "I wonder if all the kids at my school who have sex use condoms."

CORRECT ANSWER: 2

This is an age-appropriate concern, but the client's need to demonstrate that she is just like everyone else may tempt her to discontinue daily respiratory treatments and medication. The nurse should explore this statement further. Option 1: At this client's age, school commonly becomes secondary to socialization with peers. Option 3: CF would preclude this career choice, but goals can be unrealistic and changeable even among healthy children at this age. Option 4: Thoughts about sexual experimentation are common at this age. The client evidences an awareness of safe sex.

NP: Implementation
CN: Psychosocial integrity
CNS: Coping and adaptation
CL: Analysis

57 A 3-year-old boy returns from surgery with an I.V. of D_5W infusing at a rate of 40 ml/hour. How fast should the I.V. infuse when using a pediatric (mini-drip) administration set?

☐ 1. 7 gtt/minute
☐ 2. 10 gtt/minute
☐ 3. 13 gtt/minute
☐ 4. 40 gtt/minute

CORRECT ANSWER: 4
Using a pediatric administration set with a drip factor of 60 gtt/ml, the flow would be 40 gtt/minute. Options 1, 2, and 3 are flow rates of an adult administration set.
NP: Implementation
CN: Physiological integrity
CNS: Pharmacological and parenteral therapies
CL: Application

---

58 A 6-month-old male with hip dislocation has been treated for the past 6 weeks with a Frejka splint, which maintains abduction through padding of the diaper area. At his follow-up visit, the client's mother reports that she removes the splint when he gets too fussy and that he settles down and sleeps well for several hours once the extra padding is removed. Which of the following responses by the nurse is most appropriate?

☐ 1. "I can tell you are concerned about his comfort, but he must wear the padded splint except during the three times a day when you perform range-of-motion exercises on his legs."
☐ 2. "I am pleased that you recognized that the padding was too thick and adjusted it so he could sleep comfortably."
☐ 3. "I realize that seeing him uncomfortable is difficult for you, but the splint must be kept on except when you bathe him or change his diaper in order for it to help his hip."
☐ 4. "If he seems uncomfortable while wearing the splint, it is important that you call us immediately."

CORRECT ANSWER: 3
Soft abduction devices, such as the Frejka splint, must be worn continually except for diapering and skin care. Options 1 and 2: The splint is removed only for diaper care; the abduction position must be maintained to establish a deeper hip socket. Option 4: Discomfort is anticipated; appropriate responses include changing position, holding, cuddling, and providing diversions.
NP: Evaluation
CN: Physiological integrity
CNS: Physiological adaptation
CL: Application

59 A 12-year-old white male with CF wants to have three of his friends visit with him, but he is very tired and continues to lose weight in the hospital. What is the nurse's best action?

- ☐ 1. Allow the visit, as he needs to stay in contact with his peers.
- ☐ 2. Do not allow the visit, as he is too tired.
- ☐ 3. Explain his weight loss to him and suggest a telephone call to his friends instead of a visit.
- ☐ 4. Have his parents explain to him that he will be able to see his friends when he is feeling better.

CORRECT ANSWER: 3

Adolescents need to keep up with the day-to-day events of their peers. Because he is losing weight, a visit would likely overtire him. The telephone is a great way to allow him to visit with his friends without overtaxing his energy. Option 1: Allowing the visit would exhaust the client and compromise his safety. Option 2: Not allowing the visit would fail to satisfy the client's social needs and would create a negative nurse-client relationship. Option 4: Having parents explain the situation would take control away from the client.

NP: Implementation
CN: Psychosocial integrity
CNS: Coping and adaptation
CL: Application

---

60 A 13-year-old girl has been diagnosed with structural scoliosis by her school nurse. Which of the following should the nurse have the girl do to confirm the diagnosis?

- ☐ 1. Bend over and touch her toes while the nurse observes from the back.
- ☐ 2. Stand sideways while the nurse observes her profile.
- ☐ 3. Assume a knee-chest position on the examination table.
- ☐ 4. Arch her back while the nurse observes her from the front.

CORRECT ANSWER: 1

As the child bends over, the curvature of the spine is more apparent. The scapula on one side becomes more prominent, and the opposite side hollows. Options 2 and 4: Scoliosis cannot be properly assessed from the side or the front. Option 3: This is the position used for lumbar puncture.

NP: Assessment
CN: Health promotion and maintenance
CNS: Prevention and early detection of disease
CL: Comprehension

---

61 A teenage female who has suffered severe burns begins to feel better and becomes demanding of her mother's and the nurses' time. Which nursing action would be most therapeutic?

- ☐ 1. Explore with the client how the nurse can best assist in her care.
- ☐ 2. Let the client know that she must follow all hospital protocols rigidly.
- ☐ 3. Limit her use of the nurse call button to once per hour.
- ☐ 4. Encourage the client's mother to perform as much of the client's care as possible.

CORRECT ANSWER: 1

Adolescent coping behaviors are well established. Involving her in care planning can facilitate effective coping. Option 2: Adolescents need some control over their bodies and their lives. Option 3: Adolescents need to be involved in collaborative decisions regarding limit setting. Option 4: Adolescents need to be involved in collaborative decisions regarding parental care.

NP: Implementation
CN: Psychosocial integrity
CNS: Coping and adaptation
CL: Analysis

62 Which analgesic would most effectively manage a client's severe pain after suffering second- and third-degree burns?

☐ 1. Acetaminophen (Tylenol) 650 mg suppository
☐ 2. Meperidine (Demerol) 50 mg I.M.
☐ 3. Codeine 15 mg by mouth
☐ 4. Morphine 2 mg I.V.

CORRECT ANSWER: 4
A client with severe burns requires strong analgesia. The most effective method of administering analgesics is the I.V. route. Option 1: Second-degree burns are commonly too painful for acetaminophen to relieve. Option 2: I.M. medication may not be absorbed when the client is physiologically unstable. Option 3: Codeine may not provide sufficient analgesia, and oral administration is not usually the best route for severe burn victims.

NP: Implementation
CN: Physiological integrity
CNS: Pharmacological and parenteral therapies
CL: Application

---

63 A 3-year-old girl with laryngotracheal bronchitis has become restless in her croup tent. Her mother asks if she can have medication for sleep. What is the nurse's best response?

☐ 1. "I'll call her doctor for a sedative. Then she will be able to rest."
☐ 2. "You could take her out of the croup tent and rock her. That may calm her down."
☐ 3. "I'll call the physician; we may have to perform a tracheostomy."
☐ 4. "Medication for sleep could cause respiratory problems. I will assess her color, respirations, and pulse."

CORRECT ANSWER: 4
A sedative may depress the client's respirations and also may conceal the client's restlessness, a possible symptom of oxygen deprivation. Assessment of skin color, respirations, and cardiac function can determine whether hypoxia is causing the restlessness. Option 1: A sedative may further compromise the client's oxygen saturation. Option 2: Exposure to the dry room air may make breathing more difficult. Option 3: This may cause the mother much unnecessary anxiety; the data given do not indicate that such a drastic measure is indicated.

NP: Assessment
CN: Physiological integrity
CNS: Reduction of risk potential
CL: Analysis

---

64 Which of the following nursing actions can best meet the developmental needs of a 14-month-old boy who is in a private hospital room?

☐ 1. Ask the child's mother to room with the child.
☐ 2. Have nursing unit personnel visit the child regularly throughout the day.
☐ 3. Set the TV to the child's favorite cartoon shows.
☐ 4. Attach a brightly colored balloon to the child's crib.

CORRECT ANSWER: 1
The child's mother can best provide for his developmental needs by being with him all the time. At this age he is most susceptible to separation anxiety. Option 2: A child of this age is likely to be apprehensive toward unfamiliar adults. Option 3: Television is a poor substitute for human contact. Option 4: A balloon is insufficient stimulation for a child of this age.

NP: Implementation
CN: Health promotion and maintenance
CNS: Growth and development through the life span
CL: Application

65 A 9-month-old baby is admitted with acute bronchiolitis. The physician prescribes ribavirin (Virazole) via a small-particle aerosol generator. Which parameter would best indicate that the medication has produced its desired effect?

☐ 1. Wheezing is diminished.
☐ 2. Secretions are liquefied.
☐ 3. Coughing episodes increase.
☐ 4. Barrel chest is less evident.

CORRECT ANSWER: 4
Ribavirin, an antiviral agent, prohibits replication of respiratory syncytial virus, the most common cause of bronchiolitis. The hyperinflated or barrel chest, a classic sign of bronchiolitis, is caused by obstruction in the small air passages. Resolution of the virus results in decreased airway obstruction and less trapped air. Option 1: Ribavirin is not a bronchodilator. Although wheezing would diminish as the disease resolves, this would not be the best parameter to measure the drug's effectiveness. Option 2: Because ribavirin is not a mucolytic agent, liquefied secretions are not anticipated. Option 3: Paroxysms of coughing occur with bronchiolitis. Resolution of the disease would decrease, not increase, frequency.

NP: Evaluation
CN: Physiological integrity
CNS: Pharmacological and parenteral therapies
CL: Application

---

66 A client with CF performs several tasks each morning to facilitate pulmonary clearance. Which task should be done first?

☐ 1. Chest percussion and postural drainage
☐ 2. Diaphragmatic and side-bending breathing
☐ 3. Nebulization with a bronchodilator
☐ 4. One-half mile walk or jog

CORRECT ANSWER: 1
Chest percussion performed intermittently during postural drainage loosens secretions, stimulates coughing, and assists in mucus removal. Option 2: Breathing exercises are done after postural drainage and nebulization. The goal is to develop more effective diaphragmatic and intercostal breathing. Option 3: Nebulization follows postural drainage. This permits deeper penetration of droplet particles. A second episode of chest physiotherapy is optional after nebulization. Option 4: Exercise is effective in improving the client's ability to clear accumulated secretions. Recommended activities are walking, swimming, and jogging. The activity would be done after chest physiotherapy, nebulization, and breathing exercises.

NP: Implementation
CN: Physiological integrity
CNS: Physiological adaptation
CL: Application

67 The nurse is implementing a discharge teaching plan for the parents of an infant with a TEF repair. Which of the following interventions is most important?

☐ 1. Remind the parents to place the infant prone after gastrostomy feedings.
☐ 2. Instruct the parents to apply arm restraints during gastrostomy feedings.
☐ 3. Allow the parents adequate practice in doing gastrostomy feedings.
☐ 4. Advise the parents to telephone the physician daily to assess gastrostomy intake.

CORRECT ANSWER: 3
The caregiver must feel comfortable with the gastrostomy feeding, because it will be the primary source of nourishment until the client's surgical wound heals. Option 1: Infants are usually placed on their right side after feeding. Option 2: Restraints are not usually applied during gastrostomy feedings. Option 4: This would not usually be considered necessary.

NP: Implementation
CN: Safe, effective care environment
CNS: Management of care
CL: Application

---

68 An infant is admitted to the nursery from the delivery room. On initiation of the first feeding of sterile water, the infant coughs fluid through the nose and mouth, struggles for air, and turns dusky. The nurse suspects a TEF. Which assessment would be most important for the nurse to complete before telephoning the physician?

☐ 1. Maternal history of prolonged labor
☐ 2. Maternal history of hydramnios
☐ 3. Absent bowel sounds on admission to the nursery
☐ 4. Poor sucking response at initial assessment

CORRECT ANSWER: 2
A maternal history of hydramnios is linked with about 85% of infants with esophageal atresia, which is closely associated with TEF. Options 1, 3, and 4 are not associated with esophageal atresia.

NP: Assessment
CN: Health promotion and maintenance
CNS: Growth and development through the life span
CL: Comprehension

---

69 A 15-month-old female with laryngotracheobronchitis is in a mist tent. Her mother asks the nurse, "Why does she need this oxygen tent with humidity?" Which of the following would be the nurse's best response?

☐ 1. "The mist tent will control the baby's fever."
☐ 2. "It will make her feel safe in the hospital environment."
☐ 3. "It will help relieve the irritation in her airway."
☐ 4. "It is the best way to provide her with extra oxygen."

CORRECT ANSWER: 3
The purpose of the mist tent is to decrease airway irritation and edema. Option 1: Being in the mist tent may decrease the client's temperature, but this is not its primary purpose. Option 2: Because the child will be separated from her mother in the tent, she is likely to feel less than optimally secure. Option 4: If the client required only oxygen therapy, other methods of oxygen delivery could be utilized that are less restrictive of activity.

NP: Implementation
CN: Physiological integrity
CNS: Physiological adaptation
CL: Application

70 A newborn male 6 hours old has been diagnosed with esophageal atresia and TEF. On arrival at the nursery, he is placed on a radiant warming bed. Which of the following positions would be best?

☐ 1. Prone, with the head lower than the feet
☐ 2. At a 30- to 60-degree angle, with shoulders higher than hips
☐ 3. Side-lying, on the side opposite the fistula
☐ 4. Supine, with the head to the side

Correct answer: 2

This position decreases the likelihood of having gastric secretions enter the trachea. Options 1, 3, and 4 would increase the likelihood of gastric reflux into the lungs.

NP: Implementation
CN: Physiological integrity
CNS: Reduction of risk potential
CL: Application

---

71 The mother of a newborn with hypospadias tells the nurse that since her baby looks okay and can urinate, she does not see a need for corrective surgery. What is the nurse's best response?

☐ 1. "The surgery is necessary to promote a positive self-image and normal sexual function."
☐ 2. "The surgery will help your son maintain proper fluid balance and nutrition."
☐ 3. "The surgery must be done to achieve proper hormone levels and normal mobility."
☐ 4. "His sexual maturation and freedom from pain depend on the surgery."

Correct answer: 1

Objectives of surgery are to enable the child to void in the normal standing position, to improve appearance of the genitalia, and to produce a sexually adequate organ. Options 2, 3, and 4 are not relevant to problems associated with hypospadias.

NP: Implementation
CN: Physiological integrity
CNS: Reduction of risk potential
CL: Application

---

72 Which statement by the nurse will be most helpful in teaching a 14-year-old with CF about his disease?

☐ 1. "As long as you take your replacement enzymes and multivitamins, you can eat most foods."
☐ 2. "It is important for you to do your breathing exercises and postural drainage therapy at the appointed times."
☐ 3. "Even though you can have a normal sexual relationship, you may not be able to produce children."
☐ 4. "You may participate in sports activities that do not compromise your respiratory status."

Correct answer: 3

The formation of sexual relationships is a major developmental task in adolescence and must be addressed. Options 1, 2, and 4 are valid statements, but sexuality is likely to be the most pressing issue for a 14-year-old client.

NP: Implementation
CN: Health promotion and maintenance
CNS: Growth and development through the life span
CL: Analysis

73 A 6-year-old boy had rheumatic fever 3 months ago. His schoolteacher tells his mother that he has been having trouble paying attention in school since his return. Which of the following interventions would be most important for the nurse to make?

☐ 1. Observe the client's social interactions with other children in the class.
☐ 2. Watch the client for clumsiness or other neurologically based changes.
☐ 3. Keep the client away from children who sneeze or cough.
☐ 4. Test the client frequently to ensure that he has kept up with his schoolwork.

CORRECT ANSWER: 2

Sydenham's chorea, a common sequel to rheumatic fever, is commonly manifested by clumsiness, irritability, and other neurologic changes. It can occur from several weeks to several months after the initial bout of rheumatic fever. Option 1 is unnecessary; nothing in the case study indicates that the client is having a problem with social interactions. Option 3 is nearly impossible to accomplish and does not address the problem. Option 4 is inappropriate and would put undue pressure on the client.

NP: Assessment
CN: Physiological integrity
CNS: Reduction of risk potential
CL: Application

---

74 A 3-year-old client has been diagnosed with nephrotic syndrome. Which of the following would be the best nursing care goal for the client?

☐ 1. Provide rest, maintain skin integrity, and promote adequate nutritional intake.
☐ 2. Provide analgesia, maintain fluid restriction, and promote adequate rest.
☐ 3. Provide vigorous diverse activities, and promote adequate nutritional intake.
☐ 4. Promote bed rest, maintain fluid restriction, and provide analgesia.

CORRECT ANSWER: 1

Children with nephrotic syndrome are commonly lethargic and need to conserve energy. Edema requires careful attention to skin care, and anorexia requires attention to adequate nutritional intake. Options 2 and 4: Analgesia is not required in nephrotic syndrome. Option 3: Vigorous activities are not appropriate for a child with nephrotic syndrome.

NP: Planning
CN: Physiological integrity
CNS: Reduction of risk potential
CL: Application

---

75 Which of the following would be the best teaching point for a Type 1 diabetic?

☐ 1. Advise that insulin be stored at room temperature or in a cool place.
☐ 2. Encourage the client to rotate injection sites daily from thigh to abdomen to arm.
☐ 3. Emphasize that the insulin vial be shaken vigorously to mix the medication.
☐ 4. Advise that the short-acting insulin be drawn up last when two insulins are mixed.

CORRECT ANSWER: 1

Insulin should be stored in a cool place so that the protein potency is not altered. Option 2: The client should use one area (for example, the arm) for about a week and then rotate to another area, not change daily. Option 3: Insulin vials should be gently rolled to minimize the number of air bubbles created in a vial. Option 4: Short-acting insulin should be drawn up first to prevent any of the longer-acting insulin from being injected accidentally into the vial of short-acting insulin.

NP: Implementation
CN: Physiological integrity
CNS: Pharmacological and parenteral therapies
CL: Application

76 A 3-year-old girl is hospitalized with nephrosis. Which of the following morning-time assessments will be most helpful to determine if her condition is improving?

- ☐ 1. Vital signs
- ☐ 2. Daily weight
- ☐ 3. Bowel sounds
- ☐ 4. Peripheral pulses

CORRECT ANSWER: 2

Daily weight is always the best way to assess fluid status. Option 1: These are important assessment data but are not specific to nephrosis. Option 3: These are not relevant for nephrosis. Option 4: No data indicate that the evaluation of peripheral pulses would be an important part of the client's morning assessment.

NP: Evaluation
CN: Physiological integrity
CNS: Physiological adaptation
CL: Analysis

---

77 A 6-year-old girl with nephrotic syndrome is on corticosteroid therapy. Which of the following children would you choose to become her roommate?

- ☐ 1. A 3-year-old girl with cystic fibrosis who has active pneumonia
- ☐ 2. A 3-year-old boy scheduled for an open reduction of a fractured femur
- ☐ 3. A 4-year-old girl with an upper respiratory tract infection
- ☐ 4. A 5-year-old girl returning from surgery after correction of a heart defect

CORRECT ANSWER: 4

The 5-year-old has no infection and is the best match for the client in terms of age and sex. Options 1 and 3: Corticosteroids compromise the client's immune response, so she should not be placed with someone who has an active infection. Option 2: It would be better to place the client with a same-sex roommate closer to her age.

NP: Planning
CN: Safe, effective care environment
CNS: Safety and infection control
CL: Application

---

78 An infant with a surgically repaired lumbosacral myelomeningocele is now in the fifth postoperative day. Which of the following criteria would best indicate to the nurse that the client is nearly ready to go home?

- ☐ 1. Bulging fontanel
- ☐ 2. Parents visiting less frequently
- ☐ 3. No leakage from myelomeningocele sac
- ☐ 4. Weight gain

CORRECT ANSWER: 3

This normal postoperative finding indicates a successful procedure. Options 1 and 4 are signs of increasing ICP and warrant close observation. Option 2 suggests that the parents may be having trouble dealing with the child's illness. The situation must be carefully investigated before the client is discharged.

NP: Evaluation
CN: Physiological integrity
CNS: Physiological adaptation
CL: Analysis

79 A 2-year-old boy presents at the emergency department with fever, vomiting, and seizures. The results of a lumbar puncture show a high white blood cell count and a decreased glucose level. Bacterial meningitis is suspected, but the diagnosis is not yet final. Which nursing action should the nurse carry out first?

- ☐ 1. Place the client on respiratory isolation.
- ☐ 2. Complete a thorough assessment as quickly as possible.
- ☐ 3. Show the client's parents how to use the nurse's call light.
- ☐ 4. Take the client's temperature.

CORRECT ANSWER: 1

Because the most common route of spreading meningitis is via the nasopharynx, respiratory isolation should begin immediately upon admission — even before the diagnosis is confirmed. Options 2 and 4 are important, but respiratory isolation must be instituted first. Option 3 can be done later, after isolation setup and assessment are completed.

NP: Implementation
CN: Safe, effective care environment
CNS: Safety and infection control
CL: Analysis

---

80 A parent is told that her 2-year-old son has meningitis caused by *Hemophilus influenzae* and that he will be on I.V. antibiotics. The mother asks the nurse, "How long will he be on this medicine?" Which is the best response by the nurse?

- ☐ 1. 14 to 21 days
- ☐ 2. 10 to 14 days
- ☐ 3. 3 to 5 days
- ☐ 4. 4 to 7 days

CORRECT ANSWER: 2

The average length of treatment by I.V. antibiotics is 10 to 14 days, or until the child is afebrile for 5 days. Option 1: Infants usually require longer periods of treatment than older children — as much as 14 to 21 days. Options 3 and 4: These treatment durations are too short for a child of this age and condition.

NP: Implementation
CN: Physiological integrity
CNS: Pharmacological and parenteral therapies
CL: Application

---

81 What is the most appropriate site for I.M. injections for a 4-year-old child in the terminal stages of CF?

- ☐ 1. Dorsogluteal
- ☐ 2. Vastus lateralis
- ☐ 3. Deltoid
- ☐ 4. Abdomen

CORRECT ANSWER: 2

The child with terminal CF may have muscle wasting, especially in the deltoid and dorsogluteal areas. Therefore, the vastus lateralis is the best injection site. Options 1 and 3 are not good sites because of muscle wasting and potential damage to nerves. Option 4 is not an appropriate site for I.M. injections.

NP: Implementation
CN: Physiological integrity
CNS: Pharmacological and parenteral therapies
CL: Analysis

82 The nurse plans to assess a 2-year-old every hour for signs of increased ICP. Which of the following is the priority assessment?

☐ 1. Level of consciousness
☐ 2. Temperature
☐ 3. Head circumference
☐ 4. Number of stools

CORRECT ANSWER: 1
The child's level of consciousness is the most important assessment area related to changes in ICP. Option 2: Temperature should be assessed frequently during the early stages of the disease but is not needed hourly. Option 3: Head circumference is a valuable indicator of increasing ICP, but only in a child whose anterior fontanel is open. The anterior fontanel closes at 18 months. Option 4: Elimination is assessed, but hydration status, urine output, and electrolyte balance are of greater importance.

NP: Planning
CN: Physiological integrity
CNS: Physiological adaptation
CL: Analysis

---

83 A 6-month-old boy is admitted for gastroenteritis. The admitting nurse assesses him for clinical manifestations of dehydration. Which of the following findings would indicate dehydration?

☐ 1. Six wet diapers every 24 hours
☐ 2. Decreased blood pressure
☐ 3. Red, beefy tongue
☐ 4. Frequent crying

CORRECT ANSWER: 2
The child will have lower blood pressure from decreased intravascular volume. Option 1: Six wet diapers in 24 hours for a 6-month-old would not indicate fluid volume deficit. Option 3: A red, beefy tongue may be seen in contagious conditions, such as scarlet fever, or when nutritional intake is altered. Option 4: Frequent crying does not specifically suggest dehydration.

NP: Assessment
CN: Physiological integrity
CNS: Physiological adaptation
CL: Application

---

84 A 13-year-old client has received second- and third-degree burns over 40% of the body. When performing an assessment at 72 hours after the burn, the nurse should expect to find which of the following?

☐ 1. Increasing urine output
☐ 2. Severe peripheral edema
☐ 3. Respiratory distress
☐ 4. Absent bowel sounds

CORRECT ANSWER: 1
During the resuscitative-emergent phase of a burn, fluid shifts back into the interstitial space, resulting in the onset of diuresis. Option 2: Edema resolves during the emergent phase, when fluid shifts back to the intravascular space. Option 3: Respiratory rate increases during the first hours as a result of edema. When edema resolves, respirations return to normal. Option 4: Ileus occurs in the initial stage.

NP: Assessment
CN: Physiological integrity
CNS: Physiological adaptation
CL: Analysis

85 In conducting a home visit, the public health nurse notes that the mother of a toddler has cleaning materials stored beneath her kitchen and bathroom sinks. Medicines are on a tray on the dining room buffet so that family members can "remember to take them." Which of the following would be the best nursing diagnosis to make?

- ☐ 1. Knowledge deficit related to the child's level of development
- ☐ 2. Altered family processes related to role strain
- ☐ 3. Risk for injury: poisoning, related to lack of awareness of environmental hazard
- ☐ 4. Altered parenting related to unrealistic expectations of child development

CORRECT ANSWER: 3

Based on the data provided about the environment, the toddler is clearly at risk for injury. Options 1, 2, and 4: Insufficient data exist for these diagnoses.

NP: Planning
CN: Safe, effective care environment
CNS: Safety and infection control
CL: Application

---

86 A 12-year-old female with CF began taking pancrelipase (Pancrease) at 6 months of age. Which of the following actions would best help the nurse evaluate the correct use of this medication by the client?

- ☐ 1. Ask the client to demonstrate how she uses the nebulizer.
- ☐ 2. Anticipate that the electrophoresis will reflect a value less than 40 mEq/liter.
- ☐ 3. Evaluate the client's weight gain since her last visit, and obtain a description of bowel movements.
- ☐ 4. Conduct a complete respiratory assessment, and administer pulmonary function tests.

CORRECT ANSWER: 3

Pancrelipase should be taken each time the client eats a meal or snack in order to enhance digestion. This pancreatic enzyme replaces those not produced by her own obstructed pancreatic ducts and should allow the client to derive nutritional benefits from the food she eats. Her weight gain and stools should be normal. Option 1: Pancrelipase is taken orally with meals or a snack, not used in a nebulizer. Option 2: This is a measure of chloride levels, which, although they are 2 to 5 times greater in children with CF than in nonaffected children, are not influenced by pancrelipase. Option 4: Pancrelipase has no effect on respiratory status.

NP: Evaluation
CN: Physiological integrity
CNS: Pharmacological and parenteral therapies
CL: Analysis

87 The nurse instructs the mother of a 6-month-old infant admitted for gastroenteritis regarding oral rehydration therapy. Which statement made by the mother indicates correct understanding of the therapy?

- ☐ 1. "I will give my baby the special fluid at 50 ml every 10 minutes."
- ☐ 2. "I will get him to drink a carbonated beverage."
- ☐ 3. "If he vomits the solution, I will wait 20 to 30 minutes before offering more solution."
- ☐ 4. "I will offer him a fluid of choice every 10 to 15 minutes in his favorite cup."

CORRECT ANSWER: 3

The oral rehydration solution is offered every 10 to 15 minutes in small amounts of 5 to 15 ml. If vomiting occurs, the GI system needs 20 to 30 minutes to rest so that peristalsis is not increased. Option 1: This volume is too high. Oral rehydration solutions should be offered in amounts of 5 to 15 ml. Option 2: Carbonated beverages and fruit juices are contraindicated as oral rehydration solutions because their high glucose and osmolar load may stimulate additional episodes of diarrhea. Option 4: The child does not sufficiently understand his condition to select an appropriate solution.

NP: Evaluation
CN: Physiological integrity
CNS: Pharmacological and parenteral therapies
CL: Analysis

---

88 A 9-month-old girl is admitted with acute bronchiolitis. Her weight is 8 kg (17.6 lb), and respiratory rate is 60 to 70 breaths/minute. All of the following orders are written by the physician when she is admitted. Which order should the nurse question?

- ☐ 1. NPO
- ☐ 2. 1,000 ml 5% dextrose in 0.3% normal saline solution every 8 hours
- ☐ 3. Calculate urine output by weighing all wet diapers.
- ☐ 4. PPD vaccination today; record reaction 48 and 72 hours after administration.

CORRECT ANSWER: 2

Although infants have a higher fluid requirement than adults, this order, if implemented, would result in a fatal fluid overload. Infants require 125 to 145 ml/kg in 24 hours, or a maximum of 1,160 ml for this client. Administering 3,000 ml in 24 hours would give her almost three times the recommended limit. In addition, fluids are administered sparingly to patients with bronchiolitis to prevent pulmonary edema and fluid overload, so the nurse would expect less than the maximum volume to be given. Option 1: Fluids by mouth are contraindicated because of tachypnea. Option 3: Diapers are weighed before and after each voiding. The difference, in grams, is equal to the volume of urine in cubic centimeters. Option 4: The only contraindication to PPD is that it must be given before or the same day as the measles vaccine, because the measles vaccine will suppress tuberculin reactivity and can cause a false-negative reading. MMR is normally given at 15 months. Because the client is only 9 months old, the nurse would not expect her to have received the vaccine.

NP: Implementation
CN: Physiological integrity
CNS: Pharmacological and parenteral therapies
CL: Analysis

89 A 9-year-old boy with Type 1 diabetes visits the clinic. Which of the following would best ensure responsible insulin administration?

☐ 1. The client observes his parents as they administer his injection.
☐ 2. The client learns to draw up his insulin but does not inject it.
☐ 3. The client learns to administer his insulin with supervision.
☐ 4. The client manages his insulin administration independently.

CORRECT ANSWER: 3
School-age children can administer their own insulin, but supervision is needed to ensure correct procedure and dosage. Options 1 and 2 give the client too little responsibility. Option 4 gives him too much responsibility.
NP: Planning
CN: Health promotion and maintenance
CNS: Growth and development through the life span
CL: Application

---

90 Which of the following statements by the mother of an 8-year-old girl indicates correct understanding of glycosylated hemoglobin assessment?

☐ 1. "The test will be inaccurate if she ate candy yesterday."
☐ 2. "The test replaces home blood glucose monitoring."
☐ 3. "The test assesses a type of anemia acquired by Type 1 diabetics."
☐ 4. "The test gives an average blood glucose level for her over the last 3 months."

CORRECT ANSWER: 4
Glycosylated hemoglobin assessment measures RBCs with glucose molecules attached. Because the life span of a RBC is about 3 months and the glucose remains attached until the cell dies, the test is an average of the blood glucose level over 3 months. Option 1: One day's intake does not determine the test result. Option 2: The goal of the test is to assess long-term control, not to determine the blood glucose level at one point in time. Option 3: The test is not for anemia.
NP: Evaluation
CN: Physiological integrity
CNS: Reduction of risk potential
CL: Application

---

91 Which feeding plan would be best for a 3-year-old boy with nephrotic syndrome?

☐ 1. Allow the client to eat when he feels like it because of his developmental age.
☐ 2. Provide small, frequent meals high in carbohydrates and fat.
☐ 3. Provide small, frequent meals and liquids or high-protein milkshakes.
☐ 4. Keep mealtimes the same to decrease the client's anxiety over his illness.

CORRECT ANSWER: 3
A child with nephrotic syndrome is commonly lethargic and anorexic. Small, nourishing meals will be the most beneficial. Option 1: His developmental age has nothing to do with his anorexia. Option 2: A high-fat meal would exacerbate the client's hyperlipidemia. Option 4: The client is not anxious but rather anorexic.
NP: Planning
CN: Physiological integrity
CNS: Basic care and comfort
CL: Application

92 An LPN prepares to administer DPT vaccine to a 6-month-old client. Which statement by the nurse indicates a lack of understanding of the appropriate technique?

- ☐ 1. "It is necessary to wear gloves when I give the injection."
- ☐ 2. "The angle of the needle should be perpendicular to the skin."
- ☐ 3. "I will use a 25G, $^1/_2$-inch needle."
- ☐ 4. "The gluteal muscle will be the best site."

CORRECT ANSWER: 4

The preferred site for infants is the vastus lateralis. The gluteal site can be used only after the muscle has developed with locomotion. Option 1: Because contact with blood is anticipated, gloves must be worn. Option 2: An I.M.injection is given at a right angle. Option 3: 25G to 21G needles with a length of $^1/_2$ to 1 inch are recommended for children.

NP: Assessment
CN: Physiological integrity
CNS: Pharmacological and parenteral therapies
CL: Analysis

---

93 If parents or legal guardians are not available to give consent for treatment of a life-threatening situation in a minor child, which of the following statements is most accurate?

- ☐ 1. Consent may be obtained from a neighbor or close friend of the family.
- ☐ 2. Consent may not be needed in a life-threatening situation.
- ☐ 3. Consent must be in the form of a signed document; therefore, parents or guardians must be contacted.
- ☐ 4. Consent may be given by the family physician.

CORRECT ANSWER: 2

In emergencies, including danger to life or possibility of permanent injury, consent may be implied, according to the law. Options 1 and 4: Parents have full responsibility for the minor child and are required to give informed consent whenever possible. Option 3: Verbal consent may be obtained.

NP: Implementation
CN: Safe, effective care environment
CNS: Management of care
CL: Analysis

---

94 A $3^1/_2$-year-old child is admitted to the pediatric unit with a diagnosis of abdominal pain. The client is afebrile and not complaining of pain at this time. Which of the following would be most important to include in the care plan?

- ☐ 1. Feed and dress the client each day.
- ☐ 2. Advise the client's parents to go home at night so they will be fresh during the day.
- ☐ 3. Each morning, explain to the client everything that will happen that day.
- ☐ 4. Role-play with the client just before doing procedures.

CORRECT ANSWER: 4

Concrete thinking is developed in the preschool years, and learning depends primarily on the senses. Preschoolers take things literally and must receive honest and concrete information. Option 1: Preschoolers cherish independence and will want to do these tasks for themselves. Option 2: If possible, the primary caregiver should room in with the client to decrease fears and maintain as much normalcy as possible. Anxiety may cause night terrors. Option 3: Preschoolers cannot comprehend a full day's activities. They understand time best in relation to immediate activities and should be given information just before the event.

NP: Planning
CN: Health promotion and maintenance
CNS: Growth and development through the life span
CL: Analysis

95 A 3-year-old boy weighing 33 lb is hospitalized with nephrosis. He is on bed rest and a general diet with no added salt. He is taking prednisone at a prescribed daily dosage of 2 mg/kg of body weight. How much prednisone should he receive in 24 hours?

☐ 1. 15 mg
☐ 2. 30 mg
☐ 3. 50 mg
☐ 4. 60 mg

CORRECT ANSWER: 2
Because 1 kg equals about 2.2 lb, the client's weight of 33 lb is equivalent to 15 kg. The child's daily dosage is 2 mg times his weight in kilograms; in this example, 2 mg times 15 kg, which gives a 24-hour dosage of 30 mg. Options 1, 3, and 4 are inaccurate dosages based on the data given.

NP: Planning
CN: Physiological integrity
CNS: Pharmacological and parenteral therapies
CL: Analysis

---

96 The parents of a 3-year-old express concern to the nurse that their child has never had any immunizations. What is the nurse's best response?

☐ 1. "Double the number of shots will be needed now because your child is no longer an infant."
☐ 2. "Immunizations can be postponed without harm until your child enters nursery school."
☐ 3. "Immunizations are contraindicated at your child's age."
☐ 4. "The same immunizations are given until 6 years of age."

CORRECT ANSWER: 4
The American Academy of Pediatrics recommends the same sequence of immunizations, even if the original schedule was missed, until the age of 6. Option 1: The timing of immunization must be adjusted, not the number of shots. Option 2: Missed immunizations should be given as soon as possible. Option 3: Immunizations are indicated up to age 6.

NP: Planning
CN: Health promotion and maintenance
CNS: Prevention and early detection of disease
CL: Application

---

97 A 2-year-old boy has been on your nursing unit for 4 days. He has become increasingly anxious and is now throwing a temper tantrum. What is the best action for you to take?

☐ 1. Spank the child.
☐ 2. Reason with him in a firm way.
☐ 3. Ignore his outburst.
☐ 4. Threaten him with punishment.

CORRECT ANSWER: 3
A child in the middle of a temper tantrum is incapable of reasoning. Ignoring his behavior and removing anything that could injure him is the best action. Option 1: Spanking would raise his anxiety and increase his insecurity. Options 2 and 4: Threats and discussions are not effective because of his inability to listen.

NP: Implementation
CN: Health promotion and maintenance
CNS: Growth and development through the life span
CL: Application

98 What principle would the nurse use in teaching parents what to expect as their new baby begins to grow and develop?

- ☐ 1. Development proceeds in a cephalocaudal direction.
- ☐ 2. Development proceeds in a proximal-distal direction.
- ☐ 3. Development progresses from the simple to the complex.
- ☐ 4. Development is from the general to the specific.

CORRECT ANSWER: 1

Human development proceeds in a cephalocaudal direction; that is, from head to toe.

NP: Assessment
CN: Health promotion and maintenance
CNS: Growth and development through the life span
CL: Analysis

---

99 A 7-year-old boy with Type 1 diabetes takes a mixture of regular and NPH insulin. His mother asks the nurse about his participation in a weekend camping trip. What is the best nursing response?

- ☐ 1. "He should have a light snack before doing any hiking."
- ☐ 2. "He should not go on this trip. It is potentially dangerous."
- ☐ 3. "Have him increase his morning NPH insulin to compensate for higher metabolism during any hiking."
- ☐ 4. "He needs to understand the physical limitations placed on a diabetic."

CORRECT ANSWER: 1

A light meal before rigorous exercise will give the client adequate blood glucose levels during the peak action of his morning NPH insulin. Options 2 and 4 discourage the promotion of a normal lifestyle. Option 3 would increase the likelihood of a hypoglycemic reaction.

NP: Planning
CN: Physiological integrity
CNS: Reduction of risk potential
CL: Application

---

100 The nurse has just told a client that his tuberculin skin test is positive. Which of the following best shows that the client understands the test results?

- ☐ 1. "I have been exposed to tuberculosis."
- ☐ 2. "I am immune to tuberculosis and cannot catch it."
- ☐ 3. "I have a contagious stage of tuberculosis."
- ☐ 4. "I have gotten the disease back after it was cured."

CORRECT ANSWER: 1

The client has been exposed to the tubercle bacillus at some time in the past. Options 2, 3 and 4: A positive skin test does not indicate active tuberculosis, immunity, or recurrence.

NP: Evaluation
CN: Health promotion and maintenance
CNS: Prevention and early detection of disease
CL: Analysis

101 A teenage girl has been sexually abused by a family member for several years. She is now 9 weeks pregnant. While being assessed at the clinic, she asks the nurse, "What do you think I should do about being pregnant?" What is the nurse's best response?

- ☐ 1. "At your age, you stand a very good chance of having a spontaneous miscarriage."
- ☐ 2. "Only you and your mother can decide what to do about this pregnancy."
- ☐ 3. "I believe it would be all right to have an abortion at this stage of your pregnancy. Do you want that?"
- ☐ 4. "It is very hard to make the correct decision. How do you feel about being pregnant?"

CORRECT ANSWER: 4

Asking how the client feels about the situation opens up the opportunity to elicit more information. This helps the client to explore all possible options before making a decision. Option 1 is nonsupportive. Option 2 is evasive. Option 3 offers a personal opinion and inappropriately puts the nurse in command of the situation.

NP: Planning
CN: Psychosocial integrity
CNS: Coping and adaptation
CL: Analysis

---

102 You are admitting a 15-month-old boy who has bilateral otitis media and bacterial meningitis. Which is the best room for this client?

- ☐ 1. In isolation off a side hallway
- ☐ 2. A private room near the nurses' station
- ☐ 3. A room with another child who also has meningitis
- ☐ 4. A room with two toddlers who have the croup

CORRECT ANSWER: 2

With meningitis, the child should be isolated for the first day but be close to where he can be observed frequently. Option 1 is too far away for frequent observation. Options 3 and 4 would present an infectious hazard to the other children.

NP: Planning
CN: Safe, effective care environment
CNS: Management of care
CL: Analysis

Adult Nursing

1 A client with a history of renal calculi has progressively lost renal function and is admitted to the unit with a diagnosis of chronic renal failure. The physician has prescribed polystyrene sulfonate (Kayexalate). Which of the following is the best reason to use this drug in renal failure?

☐ 1. To lower serum phosphate levels
☐ 2. To correct acidosis
☐ 3. To exchange potassium for sodium
☐ 4. To prevent constipation from sorbitol use

CORRECT ANSWER: 3
In renal failure, clients become hyperkalemic because they cannot excrete potassium in urine. Polystyrene sulfonate provides the mechanism for potassium excretion by pulling potassium into the bowels and exchanging it for sodium. The potassium is then excreted in the feces. Option 1: Phosphate binders, such as aluminum hydroxide gel, are given to lower phosphate levels. Option 2: Diet changes, sodium bicarbonate, or dialysis might be used to help control acidosis. Option 4: Polystyrene sulfonate is itself constipating and must be given with a laxative such as sorbitol.

NP: Evaluation
CN: Physiological integrity
CNS: Pharmacological and parenteral therapies
CL: Application

---

2 The nurse is caring for a client who has had a scleral buckling for a detached retina. Which finding on the first postoperative day should the nurse immediately report to the physician?

☐ 1. A white blood cell (WBC) count of 6,000/µl
☐ 2. A hemoglobin level of 14 g/dl
☐ 3. Sudden onset of nausea with vomiting
☐ 4. Dizziness when sitting at the bedside

CORRECT ANSWER: 3
Nausea and vomiting may indicate increased intraocular pressure (IOP), which could result in visual loss if untreated. Vomiting also needs immediate treatment because it can contribute to increased IOP. Option 1: The WBC count is within normal range. Option 2: The hemoglobin level is within normal limits. Option 4: Dizziness on the first postoperative day is to be anticipated.

NP: Evaluation
CN: Physiological integrity
CNS: Reduction of risk potential
CL: Analysis

3 A client has end-stage renal disease (ESRD). With the azotemia, fluid accumulation, and hypertension that develop with ESRD, which nursing diagnosis would be best?

☐ 1. Risk for injury
☐ 2. Risk for infection
☐ 3. Social isolation
☐ 4. Risk for activity intolerance

CORRECT ANSWER: 1

Azotemia may lead to confusion and impaired decision making; fluid accumulation and hypertension can lead to visual changes. These changes make it necessary to assess the environment for the risk for injury. Option 2: The risk for infection is certainly a possibility for this client, but it is not specific to the signs described. Options 3 and 4: Because the client is acutely ill, social isolation and a high degree of activity intolerance would be expected; however, they are not specific to the signs described.

NP: Planning
CN: Physiological integrity
CNS: Physiological adaptation
CL: Application

---

4 A 65-year-old woman recently noted a lump in her right breast. After a needle biopsy of the lump, she was diagnosed as having a malignant breast tumor. She is scheduled to have a right-sided modified radical mastectomy tomorrow. Which statement by the client best indicates her understanding of preoperative mastectomy teaching?

☐ 1. "This surgery will surely cure my cancer."
☐ 2. "From now on I should wear gloves when gardening."
☐ 3. "I should not stretch or exercise my right arm until the incision heals."
☐ 4. "Do you think my husband will still find me attractive?"

CORRECT ANSWER: 2

Clients who have had a modified radical mastectomy have a lifelong risk of infection in the arm and hand on the side of the surgery. Measures to prevent infection include protecting the affected limb against injury. Option 1: Although surgery may cure breast cancer, it is not guaranteed. Option 3: Exercise to the affected arm usually begins within 24 hours of surgery. Option 4: Although the client's concern about her husband's feelings are legitimate, the question does not involve a teaching issue.

NP: Evaluation
CN: Physiological integrity
CNS: Reduction of risk potential
CL: Analysis

---

5 A team leader assigns tasks to a nurse's aide. Which of the following criteria is most important to consider when delegating responsibility?

☐ 1. Appropriateness of assignment
☐ 2. Learning needs of the team member
☐ 3. Team member preference
☐ 4. Compatibility of team member and client

CORRECT ANSWER: 1

The two major criteria to consider when delegating responsibility are the appropriateness and fairness of the assignment. Options 2 and 3 may lead to inappropriate assignments. Option 4 is unrealistic; health care workers must learn to care for a diverse group of clients from various socioeconomic and ethnic backgrounds.

NP: Planning
CN: Safe, effective care environment
CNS: Management of care
CL: Analysis

6 A male client who has had spinal anesthesia is under the physician's orders to lie flat postoperatively. When the client asks to go to the bathroom, the nurse encourages him to comply with the order. By complying, the client can avoid which of the following?

☐ 1. Hypotension
☐ 2. Respiratory depression
☐ 3. Headache
☐ 4. Pain at the lumbar injection site

CORRECT ANSWER: 3
Lying flat reduces the risk of headache after spinal anesthesia. Options 1 and 2: Hypotension and respiratory depression may be adverse effects of spinal anesthesia associated with the spread of the anesthetic, but lying flat is not aimed at helping to reduce these effects. Option 4: Pain at the lumbar injection site is not typically a problem.

NP: Implementation
CN: Physiological integrity
CNS: Pharmacological and parenteral therapies
CL: Application

---

7 A client scheduled for eye surgery is given one drop of phenylephrine hydrochloride (Neo-Synephrine), 2.5% solution, every 30 to 60 minutes before surgery as ordered. Which of the following outcomes should the nurse expect the drug to provide?

☐ 1. Inhibit dilation of the pupil
☐ 2. Cause pupillary constriction to decrease IOP
☐ 3. Decrease production of aqueous humor
☐ 4. Cause pupil dilation

CORRECT ANSWER: 4
Phenylephrine hydrochloride is a sympathomimetic drug used to cause mydriasis (pupillary dilation) in order to facilitate viewing of the retina. Options 1 and 2: The drug causes pupillary dilation, which can increase IOP in certain conditions. Option 3: The drug does not affect aqueous humor production.

NP: Evaluation
CN: Physiological integrity
CNS: Pharmacological and parenteral therapies
CL: Analysis

---

8 You are participating in a cancer-screening program for colorectal cancer. Which of the following clients presents the fewest risk factors for colon cancer?

☐ 1. A 45-year-old woman with a 25-year history of ulcerative colitis
☐ 2. A 50-year-old man with a father who died of colon cancer
☐ 3. A 60-year-old man who follows a diet low in fat and high in fiber
☐ 4. A 72-year-old woman with a history of breast cancer

CORRECT ANSWER: 3
Although the man is over age 40, he follows an appropriate diet and does not present other common risk factors. Option 1: Inflammatory bowel disease of long duration is a risk factor for colorectal cancer. Option 2: A family history of colon cancer is a risk factor for colorectal cancer. Option 4: Advanced age as well as breast cancer increase the risk of colorectal cancer.

NP: Assessment
CN: Health promotion and maintenance
CNS: Prevention and early detection of disease
CL: Application

9 A client diagnosed with breast cancer is receiving external radiation therapy. Which of the following self-care instructions would be most important for the nurse to provide?

- ☐ 1. Wear a tight bra to promote maximum support to the left breast.
- ☐ 2. Clean around the port site with tepid water.
- ☐ 3. Facilitate healing by exposing the radiation area to sunlight.
- ☐ 4. Use perfumed deodorant powder to promote a sense of well-being.

CORRECT ANSWER: 2
Markings of the radiation site must be retained, and neither hot nor cold temperatures should contact the skin. Option 1: Restrictive clothing should be avoided. Option 3: The potentially dry skin of the radiation site should not be exposed to the sun. Option 4: Perfumes and powders should be avoided to prevent skin drying and irritation.

NP: Planning
CN: Safe, effective care environment
CNS: Safety and infection control
CL: Application

---

10 A 55-year-old female with autoimmune Addison's disease has been admitted to your nursing unit with dehydration. Your initial assessment confirms a nursing diagnosis of fluid volume deficit. Which of the following etiologic factors establishes this nursing diagnosis?

- ☐ 1. Glucocorticoid excess
- ☐ 2. Mineralocorticoid deficiency
- ☐ 3. Melanocyte-stimulating hormone excess
- ☐ 4. Melanocyte-stimulating hormone deficit

CORRECT ANSWER: 2
Mineralocorticoid deficiency in Addison's disease causes increased losses of sodium, chloride, water, and potassium in urine, which leads to a fluid volume deficit. Option 1: Addison's disease is associated with a glucocorticoid deficit. Option 3: Melanocyte-stimulating hormone excess does not cause fluid volume deficit. Option 4: Addison's disease is characterized by a melanocyte-stimulating hormone excess.

NP: Planning
CN: Physiological integrity
CNS: Physiological adaptation
CL: Analysis

---

11 Which of the following must the nurse include in the teaching plan for a client on replacement doses of glucocorticoids?

- ☐ 1. Make up a missed dose the next time.
- ☐ 2. Take the dose with meals or snacks.
- ☐ 3. Take two-thirds of the dose in the evening.
- ☐ 4. Monitor for signs that the dosage should be increased, including weight gain, moon face, and edema.

CORRECT ANSWER: 2
The client should take glucocorticoids with meals or snacks to decrease the potential for gastric irritation. Option 1: The nurse should strongly emphasize that doses must not be omitted. Option 3: Two-thirds of the dose should be taken in the early morning. Option 4: Weight gain, moon face, and edema, all signs of Cushing's syndrome, may indicate excessive levels and are adverse effects of the drugs.

NP: Planning
CN: Physiological integrity
CNS: Pharmacological and parenteral therapies
CL: Application

12 A client arrives in the operating room appearing relaxed and drowsy. He received 75 mg of meperidine (Demerol) and 0.4 mg of atropine I.M. 1 hour ago. When you begin your assessment, the client begins talking rapidly, commenting, "I thought I'd be relaxed. Instead, I'm nervous and scared about the operation." Which of the following should the nurse do next?

- ☐ 1. The client is experiencing anxiety; listen attentively and provide realistic verbal reassurance.
- ☐ 2. The client is experiencing an adverse effect of the meperidine; report it to the physician.
- ☐ 3. The client is typically anxious; proceed with the assessment and preparation for surgery.
- ☐ 4. The client needs additional sedation; request an order from the anesthesiologist.

CORRECT ANSWER: 1

Clients routinely experience preoperative anxiety. Nurses should use basic communication skills to reduce the apprehension. Option 2: Clients do not typically experience nervousness as an adverse effect of meperidine. Option 3: This does not address the client's anxiety. Option 4: Supportive communication techniques may reduce the client's anxiety without the need for additional drugs.

NP: Planning
CN: Psychosocial integrity
CNS: Coping and adaptation
CL: Analysis

---

13 Which of the following nursing measures would be inappropriate to include when planning care for a client receiving chemotherapy via a venous access device?

- ☐ 1. Clean the insertion site and change the dressing within 24 to 72 hours.
- ☐ 2. Periodically flush the catheter with heparin.
- ☐ 3. Monitor for redness, drainage, and swelling at the insertion site.
- ☐ 4. Rotate the insertion site every 72 hours.

CORRECT ANSWER: 4

Venous access devices are commonly used for clients receiving long-term chemotherapy, total parenteral nutrition, or frequent medication or fluids. These devices may remain in place for several weeks to more than 1 year if no complications develop. Option 1: This helps prevent infection at the insertion site. Option 2: This helps prevent catheter occlusion from a thrombosis. Option 3: Monitoring is appropriate because these signs may indicate an infection at the insertion site.

NP: Planning
CN: Physiological integrity
CNS: Pharmacological and parenteral therapies
CL: Application

14 After a laminectomy, a male client has a palpable bladder and complains of lower abdominal discomfort. He is voiding 30 to 50 ml of urine at frequent intervals. Which of the following would be the best nursing intervention?

☐ 1. Observe for worsening discomfort.
☐ 2. Administer the prescribed analgesic.
☐ 3. Obtain an order for urinary catheterization.
☐ 4. Reassure the client that this is a normal voiding pattern.

CORRECT ANSWER: 3

The client has "overflow retention." A catheter relieves the discomfort by draining urine from the bladder. Option 1: Permitting further distention could injure the bladder. Option 2: Although an analgesic may relieve the discomfort, it will not resolve the cause. Option 4: Overflow retention is not normal.

NP: Planning
CN: Physiological integrity
CNS: Reduction of risk potential
CL: Application

---

15 A 62-year-old male client had drainage of a pelvic abscess secondary to diverticulitis 6 days ago. While drinking water, he begins to cough violently. His daughter runs to the nurse's station, screaming that her father has exploded. Upon entering the room, the nurse observes that the client's wound has ruptured and a small segment of bowel is protruding. What should the nurse do first?

☐ 1. Ask the client what has occurred, call the physician, have the daughter stay with her father, and cover the area with the bedsheet soaked in water.
☐ 2. Have a nursing assistant hold the wound together while you obtain the vital signs, call the physician, and flex the client's knees.
☐ 3. Obtain vital signs, call the physician, obtain emergency orders, and explain to the daughter exactly what has occurred.
☐ 4. Have the physician called while you remain with the client, flex the client's knees, and cover the wound with sterile towels soaked in sterile saline.

CORRECT ANSWER: 4

This is an emergency situation: The physician must be notified, but further injury must be prevented immediately by flexing the knees and moistening the area with sterile towels and sterile saline. The moistening prevents drying out the intestines, which could lead to necrosis, and reduces the chance of infection. Option 1: The nurse should not waste time finding out how the incident occurred. The bedsheet and water are not appropriate to use because they are not sterile. Option 2: The wound needs to be covered with sterile saline rather than just held together. Option 3: This does not include the key actions of flexing the client's knees and covering the wound with sterile towels soaked in saline.

NP: Implementation
CN: Physiological integrity
CNS: Physiological adaptation
CL: Application

16 A client has severe pruritus from hepatitis B. Which of the following nursing measures would best enhance the client's comfort?

- ☐ 1. Use hot water to increase vasodilation.
- ☐ 2. Use cold water to decrease itching sensation.
- ☐ 3. Give tepid water baths.
- ☐ 4. Avoid lotions and creams.

CORRECT ANSWER: 3

Measures to treat pruritus include tepid sponge baths and the use of emollient creams and lotions. Option 1: Hot water should be avoided because capillary dilation may increase pruritus. Option 2: Warm water is preferred to cold. Option 4: The use of emollient creams and lotions on dry skin is recommended.

NP: Implementation
CN: Physiological integrity
CNS: Basic care and comfort
CL: Application

---

17 A male client has consulted his physician with complaints of flulike symptoms off and on over the past 2 months. A blood test reveals that he is HIV-positive. The client asks the nurse when he can expect to develop acquired immunodeficiency syndrome (AIDS). Which of the following would provide the most accurate information to the client?

- ☐ 1. "When the enzyme-linked immunosorbent assay (ELISA) test results are abnormal"
- ☐ 2. "When the Western blot test results are abnormal"
- ☐ 3. "When an opportunistic infection is diagnosed"
- ☐ 4. "When seroconversion takes place"

CORRECT ANSWER: 3

AIDS is not diagnosed until an opportunistic infection is present. Options 1 and 2: The ELISA is a screening test used to detect the presence of HIV antibodies. Because the ELISA test can give false-positive results, the more expensive and specific Western blot test is used to confirm the presence of HIV antibodies. These tests together establish that the person is HIV-positive but not that the person has AIDS. Option 4: Seroconversion means that a person has gone from HIV-negative to HIV-positive.

NP: Assessment
CN: Physiological integrity
CNS: Physiological adaptation
CL: Application

---

18 A dietary aide approaches the nurse and says, "I want to know who is HIV-positive on this unit. I don't go in those rooms. That is contagious." Which of the following actions by the nurse would be most appropriate?

- ☐ 1. Identify the HIV-positive clients, and assign nursing personnel to serve those trays.
- ☐ 2. Identify the HIV-positive clients, and accompany the dietary aide to those rooms.
- ☐ 3. Explain that casual contact doesn't cause HIV, and monitor that all trays are served.
- ☐ 4. Give the dietary aide gloves, explain standard precautions, and monitor tray serving.

CORRECT ANSWER: 3

Casual contact has not been identified as a mode of transmission, and seeing that all clients receive appropriate diet is a nursing responsibility. Options 1 and 2: These actions both violate client confidentiality. Option 4: Standard precautions, which include the use of latex gloves, are indicated only when the risk of contact with blood or body fluids exists. This risk would not exist for someone serving trays.

NP: Planning
CN: Safe, effective care environment
CNS: Management of care
CL: Application

19 A nurse's aide reports for duty appearing to be under the influence of alcohol. Which of the following is the best action for the nurse to take?

☐ 1. Send the aide home.
☐ 2. Tell the aide to report for work in 1 hour.
☐ 3. Report the incident to your immediate supervisor.
☐ 4. Explain that you are concerned about the aide's ability to care for clients.

CORRECT ANSWER: 3 The nurse is obliged to report the incident in view of the ethical responsibility to ensure that clients receive competent care. Options 1 and 2: These actions avoid dealing directly with the inebriation. Option 4: The concern is legitimate, but it will do nothing to resolve the immediate problem. The nurse is obliged to prevent an impaired health care worker from delivering care.

NP: Implementation
CN: Safe, effective care environment
CNS: Management of care
CL: Analysis

---

20 A client has just had a right-sided modified radical mastectomy. Which of the following nursing measures would best prevent postoperative lymphedema?

☐ 1. Massage her right arm every 4 hours for the 1st day.
☐ 2. Elevate her right arm on return from the operating room.
☐ 3. Apply elastic bandages to her right arm on return from the operating room.
☐ 4. Medicate with analgesics at least every 4 hours.

CORRECT ANSWER: 2
Elevate the client's right arm on return from the operating room. Postoperative lymphedema is caused by interruption of the lymphatic vessels. Elevating the right arm on a pillow will promote lymphatic fluid return. Option 1: Massage is not effective in preventing lymphedema. Option 3: Elastic bandages can be detrimental. Option 4: Analgesia is not related to prevention of lymphedema.

NP: Implementation
CN: Physiological integrity
CNS: Reduction of risk potential
CL: Application

---

21 A 46-year-old male client is admitted to the hospital with a suspected diagnosis of hepatitis B. He is jaundiced and is complaining of weakness. Which of the following should the nurse include in the client's plan of care?

☐ 1. Rest periods after small, frequent meals
☐ 2. A low-protein diet
☐ 3. Menus selected by the client
☐ 4. Regular exercise

CORRECT ANSWER: 1
Rest periods and small, frequent meals are necessary for clients with hepatitis B. Option 2: A diet high in protein is recommended to enhance recovery of injured liver cells. Option 3: The client needs some guidance. Choices can be made from high-protein foods. Option 4: Rest, not exercise, is indicated during the acute phase of the disease.

NP: Planning
CN: Physiological integrity
CNS: Basic care and comfort
CL: Application

22 After surgery for a bowel obstruction, a client develops acute renal failure and, 10 days later, enters the second phase of the disease. Which of the following indicates that the client has entered the second phase?

☐ 1. Urine output of less than 400 ml/day
☐ 2. Stabilization of renal function
☐ 3. Daily doubling of urine output (4 to 5 L/day)
☐ 4. Urine output of less than 100 ml/day

CORRECT ANSWER: 3
Daily doubling of urine output (4 to 5 L/day) indicates that the nephrons are healing and the client is passing into the second phase (diuresis). Option 1: Urine output of less than 400 ml/day indicates oliguria. Option 2: Renal function does not stabilize until the recovery phase (unless permanent damage has occurred, in which case it may never stabilize). Option 4: Urine output of less than 100 ml/day indicates anuria.

NP: Assessment
CN: Physiological integrity
CNS: Physiological adaptation
CL: Analysis

---

23 Which assessment finding in a client with Addison's disease would most probably warrant a nursing diagnosis of fluid volume deficit?

☐ 1. Leathery, pliable skin
☐ 2. Pretibial pitting edema
☐ 3. Pedal pulses of 4+
☐ 4. Dry skin with poor turgor

CORRECT ANSWER: 4
Fluid volume deficit is characterized by dry skin and mucous membranes, decreased skin turgor, hypotension, tachycardia, increased body temperature, and weakness. Option 1: Pliable skin is not characteristic of fluid volume deficit. Option 2: Edema may occur in some types of fluid volume deficit, but this is not a typical finding. Option 3: Fluid volume deficit reduces circulating fluid volume, leading to decreased peripheral pulses.

NP: Assessment
CN: Physiological integrity
CNS: Physiological adaptation
CL: Analysis

24 A female client is receiving doxorubicin (Adriamycin) I.V. for cancer therapy. The nurse enters her room and notes swelling and redness at the insertion site. Extravasation is confirmed. Which of the following actions should the nurse take next?

☐ 1. Slow the infusion to a keep-vein-open rate.
☐ 2. Discontinue the doxorubicin and begin an infusion of dextrose 5% in water (D_5W).
☐ 3. Discontinue the I.V. and apply ice to the site.
☐ 4. Discontinue the I.V. and inject a neutralizing solution into the area after aspirating any infiltrated drug from the tissues.

CORRECT ANSWER: 3

Vesicants, such as doxorubicin, may cause tissue necrosis and damage to underlying tendons, nerves, and blood vessels; therefore, when extravasation occurs, the I.V. infusion should be discontinued immediately. Ice constricts vessels, decreases drug absorption, and minimizes tissue injury. Option 1: Allowing the infusion to continue when extravasation has occurred increases the risk of tissue damage. Option 2: Starting an infusion of D_5W in water would not minimize tissue damage in the area of extravasation. Option 4: A physician should aspirate doxorubicin and inject a neutralizing solution when extravasation has occurred.

NP: Implementation
CN: Physiological integrity
CNS: Pharmacological and parenteral therapies
CL: Application

---

25 A client on chemotherapy has a WBC count below 1,000/µl. Which of the following nursing interventions would be most appropriate?

☐ 1. Encourage the client to keep a bowl of fresh fruit at the bedside to snack on.
☐ 2. Remove fresh flowers and potted plants from the room.
☐ 3. Avoid I.M. injections.
☐ 4. Encourage the client to walk in the hall every hour to reduce the chance of thrombus formation.

CORRECT ANSWER: 2

The water in fresh plants and the damp, moist soil in potted plants are good media for bacterial growth. Clients with a low WBC count are more susceptible to infection and should avoid exposure to these elements. Option 1: Fresh fruits and vegetables harbor bacteria not removed by ordinary washing and thus should be avoided by clients with decreased WBC counts. Option 3: I.M. injections are to be avoided in clients experiencing thrombocytopenia. Option 4: Ambulation in the hall could expose the client to other persons who are ill, thus increasing the chances of acquiring an infection; reducing the risk of thrombus formation would not affect the client's WBC count.

NP: Implementation
CN: Safe, effective care environment
CNS: Safety and infection control
CL: Application

26 A client is receiving pelvic irradiation. The nurse knows that frequent loose stools are a common adverse effect of radiotherapy to this area. Which of the following foods should the nurse recommend to the client in discharge teaching to help prevent this adverse effect?

☐ 1. Applesauce, pears, turnip greens, and fried chicken
☐ 2. Hamburger with fresh tomatoes, lettuce, carrots, and french fries
☐ 3. Sandwiches on whole wheat bread, bran cereal, and cabbage
☐ 4. Scrambled eggs, roast turkey, and bananas

CORRECT ANSWER: 4

A low-residue diet is recommended for persons experiencing diarrhea from radiotherapy. Options 1, 2, and 3: Fresh fruits, leafy green vegetables, and bran cereals are all high in residue and should be avoided.

NP: Implementation
CN: Physiological integrity
CNS: Reduction of risk potential
CL: Comprehension

---

27 After an adrenalectomy, a client receives discharge instructions for taking prescribed medication. Which statement best indicates that the client has understood the instructions?

☐ 1. "I'll only need medication for 3 months, and then I'll be back to normal."
☐ 2. "I will need to have close medical supervision for the first few months in order to adjust the medication to my needs."
☐ 3. "I will develop a full face and gain weight because of this surgery."
☐ 4. "All my problems are over, and I'll be able to do whatever I want, when I want."

CORRECT ANSWER: 2

Clients who have had an adrenalectomy must be carefully monitored to adjust the medication dosage as needed. Option 1: The client will require lifelong replacement medication. Option 3: The surgery itself will not cause weight gain or full face, but they could occur as an adverse effect of the medication. Option 4: The client will need to manage his condition carefully, especially during times of stress.

NP: Evaluation
CN: Health promotion and maintenance
CNS: Prevention and early detection of disease
CL: Analysis

---

28 A client is receiving external radiation therapy to her thoracic and lumbar spine because of metastatic breast cancer. Which of the following people should be permitted to visit?

☐ 1. Her pregnant granddaughter
☐ 2. Her husband, who is recovering from the flu
☐ 3. Her grandson and his family, including his wife and four children who are between the ages of 4 and 8
☐ 4. Her elderly sister, who has a history of chronic obstructive pulmonary disease (COPD) and frequent respiratory infections

CORRECT ANSWER: 1

The pregnant granddaughter is in no danger from external radiation therapy, and the visitor would pose no health threat to the client. Option 2: The husband should not visit until he is fully recovered from the flu because of the risk of infection. Option 3: Large crowds and children who could possibly spread upper respiratory infections should be avoided. Option 4: The sister could spread a respiratory infection.

NP: Implementation
CN: Safe, effective care environment
CNS: Safety and infection control
CL: Application

29 A 43-year-old client has started chemotherapy after having a lumpectomy for breast cancer. Alopecia is an adverse effect of one of the three drugs she is receiving. The client has long hair, which she pulls back with a barrette. The nurse assists the client with her fear about losing her hair by discussing the need to shop for an acceptable wig. Which of the following instructions should the nurse also provide?

☐ 1. Use a hair dryer, and brush after shampooing to speed drying.
☐ 2. Shampoo every other day to stimulate the hair follicles.
☐ 3. Have a permanent to eliminate the need to use a curling iron.
☐ 4. Consider cutting hair to minimize pulling and tangling.

CORRECT ANSWER: 4
Shorter hair is less susceptible to trauma and resulting hair loss. Options 1, 2, and 3: Hair dryers, frequent shampooing, and permanents all cause trauma, which might promote hair damage and loss.
NP: Planning
CN: Physiological integrity
CNS: Reduction of risk potential
CL: Application

---

30 A client receiving external radiation for metastatic cancer reports nausea and stomach upset after a week of therapy. Which of the following instructions would best ensure adequate nutritional intake?

☐ 1. Eat just before the radiation therapy.
☐ 2. Follow a high-residue, low protein, low-cholesterol diet.
☐ 3. Eat a hearty breakfast, including fruit, milk, cereal, eggs, and toast.
☐ 4. Refrain from eating for 1 hour after therapy.

CORRECT ANSWER: 3
Breakfast is usually the best tolerated meal and should contain the maximum nutritional intake. Options 1 and 4: Food should be avoided for 2 to 3 hours before and after treatment. Option 2: A high-protein, high-carbohydrate, low-residue diet is better tolerated than other diets.
NP: Planning
CN: Physiological integrity
CNS: Basic care and comfort
CL: Application

---

31 A client receiving hemodialysis treatments has had surgery to form an arteriovenous fistula. Which of the following is most important for the nurse to be aware of when providing care for the client?

☐ 1. Using a stethoscope for auscultating the fistula is contraindicated.
☐ 2. The client feels best immediately after the dialysis treatment.
☐ 3. Taking a blood pressure reading on the affected arm can cause clotting of the fistula.
☐ 4. The client should not feel pain during initiation of dialysis.

CORRECT ANSWER: 3
Pressure on the fistula or on the extremity can decrease blood flow and precipitate clotting. Option 1: Auscultation of a bruit in the fistula is one way to determine patency. Option 2: Typically, clients feel fatigued immediately after hemodialysis because of the rapid change in fluid and electrolyte status. Option 4: Although the area over the fistula may have some decreased sensation, the needle stick is still painful.
NP: Implementation
CN: Physiological integrity
CNS: Physiological adaptation
CL: Application

32 A client with diabetes mellitus has had declining renal function over the past several years. He is placed on hemodialysis because of persistently elevated creatinine levels. Which diet regimen would be best for the client on days between dialysis?

- ☐ 1. No restrictions
- ☐ 2. Low-protein diet with a prescribed amount of water
- ☐ 3. Low-protein diet with an unlimited amount of water
- ☐ 4. No protein in the diet and use of a salt substitute

CORRECT ANSWER: 2

Although dialysis removes water, creatinine, and urea from the blood, the client's diet still must be monitored. Options 1 and 3: Fluid and protein restrictions are needed. Excessive fluid intake could cause volume overload and precipitate heart failure. Excessive protein intake can produce uremic signs and symptoms, such as taste alterations, metabolic acidosis, and pruritus. Option 4: The client requires some protein to meet metabolic needs. A salt substitute should not be used without a physician's order because the product may contain potassium, and diabetic clients already tend to be hyperkalemic.

NP: Implementation
CN: Physiological integrity
CNS: Physiological adaptation
CL: Analysis

---

33 A client is being evaluated for a possible renal tumor. Which of the following assessments would be most suspicious for renal cancer?

- ☐ 1. Intermittent hematuria
- ☐ 2. Polyuria
- ☐ 3. Frothy, dark amber urine
- ☐ 4. Cloudy, foul-smelling urine

CORRECT ANSWER: 1

Intermittent hematuria is the classic sign of renal and bladder cancer. Because it is intermittent, the client may dismiss its seriousness. Option 2: Polyuria is associated with diabetes mellitus and diabetes insipidus. Option 3: Liver disease and blocked bile ducts can cause dark urine because bile cannot be excreted into the duodenum. Option 4: Cloudy, foul-smelling urine is associated with urinary tract infection.

NP: Assessment
CN: Health promotion and maintenance
CNS: Prevention and early detection of disease
CL: Analysis

34 A 36-year-old client is scheduled for a cholecystectomy this morning. Preoperative medication has been administered. While completing the preoperative checklist, the nurse discovers that the client has not signed the consent for surgery. What should the nurse do next?

☐ 1. Send the client to surgery.
☐ 2. Have the client sign the consent form now.
☐ 3. Inform the physician.
☐ 4. Have a family member sign the consent.

CORRECT ANSWER: 3
The physician has a legal obligation to obtain the client's informed consent to surgical intervention. Option 1: Except in life-threatening emergencies, surgery cannot legally be performed until consent is given. Option 2: Preoperative medication has rendered the client incompetent to sign the consent. Option 4: A client of legal age (18 years) and competency, not his family, must sign the consent for surgical treatment.

NP: Implementation
CN: Safe, effective care environment
CNS: Management of care
CL: Application

---

35 A nurse is giving a client a bed bath. The client says, "Last night someone in a white lab coat woke me up and said he wanted to get a sample of my spinal fluid. I was very sleepy and said no. Who was it and why did he want a spinal sample?" Which of the following would be the nurse's best response?

☐ 1. "You were right to send him away. It could have been anyone."
☐ 2. "I don't know who it was, but don't worry about it."
☐ 3. "Has he returned to talk to you today?"
☐ 4. "I will find out who it was and why he was here."

CORRECT ANSWER: 4
Clients have the right to know the names, qualifications, and titles of all personnel responsible for their care as well as information about their diagnostic tests and treatments. Options 1 and 2: These answers give false reassurance and do not address the client's concern. Option 3: If the person had returned to talk, the client probably would have mentioned it.

NP: Assessment
CN: Safe, effective care environment
CNS: Management of care
CL: Application

---

36 A 30-year-old teacher performs self-breast examinations monthly. Which of the following findings should she report promptly?

☐ 1. Areolae that are bilaterally darkened in color
☐ 2. Freely movable masses that become tender before the menstrual period
☐ 3. Multiple tender, round masses in both breasts
☐ 4. A hard, nontender mass in the upper outer quadrant of the left breast

CORRECT ANSWER: 4
Hard, nontender masses are associated with cancerous tumors. The upper outer quadrant is the most common site. Option 1: Darkened areolae are associated with hormonal changes, such as those caused by pregnancy. Options 2 and 3: Multiple tender, round masses in both breasts that become tender before a menstrual period indicate fibrocystic breast problems.

NP: Assessment
CN: Health promotion and maintenance
CNS: Prevention and early detection of disease
CL: Application

37 A client with Addison's disease and suspected fluid volume deficit is admitted to your unit. Vital signs on admission are temperature, 100.2°F (37.9°C); pulse, 98 beats/minute; respiratory rate, 22 breaths/minute; and blood pressure, 102/64 mm Hg. Which of the following actions should the nurse take next?

- ☐ 1. Take orthostatic vital signs.
- ☐ 2. Place the client in modified Trendelenburg's position.
- ☐ 3. Keep the client on nothing-by-mouth status.
- ☐ 4. Monitor the client for increased intracranial pressure (ICP).

CORRECT ANSWER: 1

Taking orthostatic vital signs will help determine the severity of fluid volume deficit. Option 2: There is no need at this time to place the client in modified Trendelenburg's position, which is used to counter symptoms of hypovolemic shock. Option 3: Encouraging fluid intake to restore fluid volume would be preferable. Option 4: No symptoms indicate that the client has increased ICP, which is not a typical sign of Addison's disease.

NP: Implementation
CN: Physiological integrity
CNS: Physiological adaptation
CL: Analysis

---

38 Identification of the client on admittance to the surgical suite is one of the circulating nurse's responsibilities. Which of the following is the most appropriate verification of a client's identification?

- ☐ 1. Call the client by name.
- ☐ 2. Check the surgical list and suite assignment.
- ☐ 3. Compare the arm bracelet to the chart information.
- ☐ 4. Question the orderly who brought the client.

CORRECT ANSWER: 3

Comparing the name and hospital number on the arm bracelet with the chart best verifies the client's identity. Option 1: The client may be confused and respond to a different name. Option 2: This does not ensure that the client brought into the surgical suite is the one whose name appears on the surgical list. Once the client's identity has been established, this should be cross-checked with the name on the surgical list. Option 4: The orderly could have made a mistake. The only definitive way to prevent surgery on the wrong client is to check the identity on the arm band.

NP: Assessment
CN: Safe, effective care environment
CNS: Safety and infection control
CL: Comprehension

---

39 A male client has received a combination of chemotherapy drugs for advanced cancer with brain metastasis. His platelet count is $20,000/mm^3$; hemoglobin level, 10 g/dl; and hematocrit, 42%. He is admitted for treatment of dehydration with I.V. fluids. Which of the following nursing interventions is most appropriate?

- ☐ 1. Start the I.V. with a 16G or 18G catheter.
- ☐ 2. Apply pressure on an unsuccessful venipuncture site for 2 to 3 minutes.
- ☐ 3. Administer analgesics I.M.
- ☐ 4. Wrap the I.V. site with gauze.

CORRECT ANSWER: 4

The client is prone to bleeding and needs safety precautions to protect skin integrity. Option 1: A small catheter should be used to prevent bleeding. Option 2: For a client with such a low platelet count, the nurse should apply pressure for 10 minutes or until the bleeding stops. Option 3: The nurse should avoid the I.M. route, if possible, to prevent bleeding. The oral route or I.V. route is preferable.

NP: Implementation
CN: Physiological integrity
CNS: Reduction of risk potential
CL: Application

40 A 42-year-old male complains of extreme fatigue and weakness after his 1st week of radiation therapy. Which of the following responses by the nurse would best reassure him?

☐ 1. "These symptoms usually result from radiation therapy; however, we will continue to monitor your laboratory and X-ray studies."
☐ 2. "These symptoms are part of your disease and can't be helped."
☐ 3. "Don't be concerned about these symptoms. Everybody feels this way after having radiation therapy."
☐ 4. "This is a good sign. It means that only the cancer cells are dying."

CORRECT ANSWER: 1
Fatigue and weakness result from radiation treatment and usually do not represent deterioration or disease progression. Option 2: The symptoms associated with radiation therapy usually decrease after therapy ends. Option 3: The symptoms may concern the client and should not be belittled. Option 4: Radiation destroys both cancerous and normal cells.

NP: Analysis
CN: Physiological integrity
CNS: Physiological adaptation
CL: Application

---

41 Which of the following statements best indicates that a client with hepatitis B understands the discharge teaching?

☐ 1. "My family knows that if I become tired and start vomiting, I may be getting sick again."
☐ 2. "Now I can never get hepatitis again."
☐ 3. "I'll never have a problem with my liver again, even if I drink alcohol."
☐ 4. "I can safely give blood after 3 months."

CORRECT ANSWER: 1
Hepatitis B is typically marked by reappearing signs and symptoms of fatigue, nausea, vomiting, bleeding, and bruising. Option 2: Hepatitis B can recur. Option 3: Alcohol is metabolized by the liver and should be avoided by a client with hepatitis B. Option 4: Clients who have had hepatitis are permanently barred from donating blood.

NP: Evaluation
CN: Physiological integrity
CNS: Physiological adaptation
CL: Application

---

42 A licensed practical nurse says, "The assignments are always unfair. I have the heaviest workload every day." Which of the following would be the best response by the team leader?

☐ 1. "It is not my fault. Everybody has to understand that sick clients have to be cared for."
☐ 2. "I am sorry, but I am trying to do the best I can with the staff assignments."
☐ 3. "I realize you are upset about the assignment. Let's sit down and talk about it after lunch."
☐ 4. "You are an experienced nurse on this unit. I don't feel your attitude is a good example for other staff members."

CORRECT ANSWER: 3
This is an empathetic response and indicates that the nurse is receptive to listening to the staff member's point of view. It is possible that assignments can be made more equitably; it is also possible that the "heavier workload" is only perceived. This provides a forum for discussion. Option 1: An aggressive response such as this will not resolve the conflict. Option 2: This nonassertive response eliminates exploration of solutions. Option 4: This negative response clouds the real issue that the staff member raised.

NP: Implementation
CN: Safe, effective care environment
CNS: Management of care
CL: Application

43 A female client experiences alopecia resulting from chemotherapy, prompting the nursing diagnoses of body image disturbance and self-esteem disturbance. Which of the following would best indicate that the client is meeting the goal of improved body image and self-esteem?

☐ 1. The client requests that her family bring her makeup and wig.
☐ 2. The client begins to discuss the future with her family.
☐ 3. The client reports less disruption from pain and discomfort.
☐ 4. The client cries openly when discussing her disease.

CORRECT ANSWER: 1
Requesting her wig and makeup indicates that the client with alopecia is becoming interested in looking her best and that her body image and self-esteem may be improving. Options 2, 3, and 4 may indicate that other nursing goals are being met, but they do not assess improved body image and self-esteem.
NP: Evaluation
CN: Psychosocial integrity
CNS: Coping and adaptation
CL: Analysis

---

44 A 32-year-old female is to begin chemotherapy this week on your unit. She is concerned about developing stomatitis, a complication her aunt experienced after treatment with 5-fluorouracil. Which of the following interventions would help prevent stomatitis?

☐ 1. Encourage the client to rinse her mouth with Listerine mouthwash after meals.
☐ 2. Administer a topical anesthetic, such as viscous lidocaine, before meals.
☐ 3. Use a nonabrasive toothpaste to brush teeth after meals, and floss every 24 hours.
☐ 4. Provide small, frequent feedings.

CORRECT ANSWER: 3
Frequent oral hygiene (thorough brushing after meals and flossing at least once daily) is recommended to help prevent stomatitis in the client receiving chemotherapy. Option 1: Commercial mouthwashes dry oral tissues and potentiate tissue breakdown in the oral cavity. Option 2: Administration of viscous lidocaine before meals may hasten the development of stomatitis, because the client may not feel sharp crusts or extreme food temperatures that could damage the oral mucosa. Option 4: Small, frequent feedings would not prevent stomatitis.
NP: Implementation
CN: Physiological integrity
CNS: Reduction of risk potential
CL: Application

---

45 The head nurse is orienting a new graduate nurse, who asks about caring for a client with an internal radiation implant. Which of the following would be the head nurse's best instruction?

☐ 1. Keep all linen in the room during treatment.
☐ 2. Use gloves to handle radioactive material.
☐ 3. Keep an aluminum-lined container in the room for radiation material.
☐ 4. Stand at the foot of the bed rather than the side when providing care.

CORRECT ANSWER: 1
Linens are kept in the room so that they can be examined in case radiation material dislodges. Option 2: Radiation material should only be handled by forceps, never touched with the hands. Option 3: The container for radiation material is lined with lead. Option 4: This response does not address the time, shielding, and distance principles.
NP: Planning
CN: Safe, effective care environment
CNS: Safety and infection control
CL: Application

46 After the first hemodialysis treatment, a client develops headache, hypertension, restlessness, mental confusion, nausea, and vomiting. Which of the following do these signs and symptoms indicate?

☐ 1. Peritonitis
☐ 2. Disequilibrium syndrome
☐ 3. Hypervolemia
☐ 4. Respiratory distress

CORRECT ANSWER: 2
Disequilibrium syndrome develops toward the end of or just after hemodialysis. It results when excess solutes are cleared from the blood more rapidly than they can diffuse from the body's cells into the vascular system. Options 1 and 4: Peritonitis and respiratory distress are possible complications of peritoneal dialysis. Option 3: Hypovolemia, not hypervolemia, can occur as a result of rapid fluid removal during dialysis.

NP: Assessment
CN: Physiological integrity
CNS: Physiological adaptation
CL: Analysis

---

47 An 18-year-old male has suffered a C5 spinal cord contusion that has resulted in quadriplegia. His mother is crying in the waiting room 2 days after the injury has occurred. When you sit down to talk to her, she asks whether or not her son will ever play football again. Which of the following would be your best response?

☐ 1. Reassure her that given time and motivation, he will return to normal function.
☐ 2. Advise her that it is not in his best interest for her to be so upset, and explain the importance of moral support.
☐ 3. Reflect on how she is feeling, and encourage her to express other fears that she has about his injury.
☐ 4. Explain that you are not sure, but you will call the physician to talk to her right away.

CORRECT ANSWER: 3
Listening and encouraging her to express her feelings will be most therapeutic and will allow the nurse to gather more data about the mother's understanding of the injury. Option 1: This is false reassurance; in many cases, spinal cord contusion results in permanent loss of function. Option 2: The mother needs to be allowed to voice her concerns rather than being burdened right now about giving moral support. Option 4: The physician will not be able to answer her question either; definitive prognosis is not possible so soon after a spinal cord contusion.

NP: Implementation
CN: Psychosocial integrity
CNS: Coping and adaptation
CL: Analysis

48 A 78-year-old female has been discharged recently from the hospital after experiencing heart failure related to long-standing hypertension and coronary artery disease. A community health nurse is evaluating her compliance with medication therapy. Which of the following factors best indicates that the client is complying with digoxin (Lanoxin) therapy?

☐ 1. Her ability to count her radial pulse correctly
☐ 2. Her weight gain of 2 lb in less than a week
☐ 3. An apical heart rate of 101 beats/minute
☐ 4. Absence of a pericardial friction rub

CORRECT ANSWER: 1
A client who complies with drug therapy is less likely to have a recurrence of cardiac failure. Correctly checking the radial pulse daily helps prevent a toxic reaction to digoxin. Options 2 and 3: A weight gain of 2 lb in less than 1 week and an apical heart rate greater than 100 beats/minute are signs of heart failure, possibly indicating that the client has not taken the digoxin as prescribed. Option 4: Pericardial friction rub has no relationship to digoxin therapy.

NP: Evaluation
CN: Physiological integrity
CNS: Pharmacological and parenteral therapies
CL: Analysis

---

49 A 63-year-old female client has a 10-year history of rheumatoid arthritis. Her 40-year-old daughter has recently noticed that she herself wakes up with stiff joints. The client shares her concerns about this with you. What would be the most appropriate response?

☐ 1. Explain that rheumatoid arthritis does not have a genetic basis, so there is nothing for her to be concerned about.
☐ 2. Tell her that there is some evidence that a genetic basis for the disease may exist, and suggest that the daughter be evaluated.
☐ 3. Have her suggest that her daughter take aspirin for a few days to see if the stiffness is relieved.
☐ 4. Reassure her that it is normal for a 40-year-old female to have aches and pains and that her concern is probably unwarranted.

CORRECT ANSWER: 2
Some research has indicated that a genetic link may be present. Option 1: Her concern is warranted, as there is some evidence of a genetic link. Option 3: Unexplained joint stiffness at age 40 should be evaluated by a physician before aspirin therapy is initiated on a regular basis. Option 4: There is no basis for this false reassurance.

NP: Assessment
CN: Physiological integrity
CNS: Reduction of risk potential
CL: Application

50 A client is admitted to the hospital for hip replacement surgery. Which statement by the client would indicate the need for further preoperative teaching?

☐ 1. "I will rest in bed for 2 to 3 hours after surgery."
☐ 2. "I should do muscle-strengthening exercises in both legs."
☐ 3. "I will begin gait training within 48 hours."
☐ 4. "I must turn, cough, and breathe deeply every 2 hours."

CORRECT ANSWER: 1
After total joint replacement, few clients can get up this soon, although most are out of bed within 24 hours of surgery. Options 2, 3, and 4 indicate that the client understands preoperative instructions.

NP: Evaluation
CN: Physiological integrity
CNS: Reduction of risk potential
CL: Analysis

---

51 A client is in the first postoperative day after a total laryngectomy and radical neck dissection. Which of the following is a priority goal?

☐ 1. Communicate by use of esophageal speech.
☐ 2. Improve body image and self-esteem.
☐ 3. Attain optimal levels of nutrition.
☐ 4. Maintain a patent airway.

CORRECT ANSWER: 4
Although all options are appropriate postoperative goals, maintaining a patent airway takes priority, especially on the first postoperative day. A laryngectomy tube is most likely to be in place, and suctioning is commonly needed to clear secretions. Edema and hematoma formation at the surgical site also can increase the risk of a blocked airway. Options 1 and 3 are important but would not take priority on the first postoperative day. Option 2 is a long-term goal.

NP: Planning
CN: Physiological integrity
CNS: Reduction of risk potential
CL: Analysis

---

52 A client undergoes a rhinoplasty to repair a nasal fracture in which displacement has caused an airway obstruction. Postoperatively, the client swallows frequently and requires frequent changes of the mustache dressing, which is soiled with bright red blood. Which is the best action for the nurse to take?

☐ 1. Offer the client an ice pack to decrease edema and control bleeding.
☐ 2. Offer the client a cold drink to soothe the throat.
☐ 3. Explain to the client that a tube was in the throat for the anesthetic.
☐ 4. Check the pharynx with a penlight for bleeding, and notify the physician.

CORRECT ANSWER: 4
Repeated swallowing after a rhinoplasty is a sign of postnasal bleeding; the physician should be notified. Options 1 and 2: Neither an ice pack nor a cold drink will control the bleeding. Option 3: Rhinoplasty is performed under a local, not general, anesthetic, so an endotracheal tube is not used.

NP: Assessment
CN: Physiological integrity
CNS: Physiological adaptation
CL: Analysis

53 The nurse is teaching a female client with osteoporosis about her prescribed diet. Which of the following foods is the best source of calcium?

☐ 1. 1 cup of low-fat yogurt
☐ 2. 1 cup of skim milk
☐ 3. 1 oz of cheddar cheese
☐ 4. 1 cup of ice cream

Correct answer: 1
One cup of low-fat yogurt contains 415 mg of calcium. Option 2: One cup of skim milk has 302 mg of calcium. Option 3: One ounce of cheddar cheese has 20 mg of calcium. Option 4: One cup of ice cream has 176 mg of calcium.
NP: Planning
CN: Physiological integrity
CNS: Basic care and comfort
CL: Application

---

54 An 83-year-old female client arrives at the emergency department (ED) after falling on the ice outside her senior citizens' housing facility. The admitting diagnosis is right hip fracture. Which of the following would be most important for the nurse to assess?

☐ 1. Leg shortening
☐ 2. Complaints of pain
☐ 3. Neurovascular compromise
☐ 4. Internal or external rotation

Correct answer: 3
Because impaired circulation can cause permanent damage, neurovascular assessment of the affected leg is always a priority assessment. Options 1 and 4: Leg shortening and internal or external rotation are common findings with a fractured hip. Option 2: Pain, especially on movement, is also common after a hip fracture.
NP: Assessment
CN: Physiological integrity
CNS: Reduction of risk potential
CL: Application

---

55 A client has a Hoffman apparatus on a fractured leg, using an external device with pins to fixate the fracture. One of the physician's postoperative orders reads, "Pin care every shift." What should the nurse do to implement the order?

☐ 1. Turn the pins of the Hoffman device each shift.
☐ 2. Clean the skin areas where the pins enter the client's leg each shift.
☐ 3. Soak the affected leg and Hoffman device each shift to clean the pins.
☐ 4. Remove the pins from the device, clean the pins, and replace them each shift.

Correct answer: 2
Pin care involves cleaning the skin around the pins of the Hoffman device and may include applying antimicrobial ointment. Options 1 and 4: Only a physician may manipulate the Hoffman apparatus. Option 3: The leg and apparatus should not be soaked.
NP: Implementation
CN: Physiological integrity
CNS: Physiological adaptation
CL: Analysis

56 Which of the following choices would best provide a diet high in iron for a client with anemia?

- ☐ 1. Scrambled eggs, orange juice, coffee cake, milk, and tea
- ☐ 2. Poached eggs, melon, toast, apple juice, and coffee
- ☐ 3. Oatmeal, milk, toast, an orange, and coffee
- ☐ 4. Fortified cereal, dried peach halves, orange juice, and hot chocolate

CORRECT ANSWER: 4

Whole grain and enriched breads and cereals are higher in iron than are refined, unenriched breads and cereals. Options 1, 2, and 3: Milk is a poor source of iron; tea and coffee inhibit iron absorption.

NP: Planning
CN: Physiological integrity
CNS: Basic care and comfort
CL: Application

---

57 During afternoon rounds, the nurse finds a male client using a pencil to scratch inside his knee-to-toe cast. The client is complaining of severe itching in the ankle area. Which action should the nurse take?

- ☐ 1. Allow him to continue to scratch inside the cast with a pencil.
- ☐ 2. Give him a sterile metal object to use for scratching instead of the pencil.
- ☐ 3. Encourage him to avoid scratching, and obtain an order for diphenhydramine (Benadryl) if severe itching persists.
- ☐ 4. Obtain an order for a sedative, such as diazepam (Valium), to prevent him from scratching.

CORRECT ANSWER: 3

Most clients can be discouraged from scratching if given a mild antihistamine, such as diphenhydramine, to relieve itching. Options 1 and 2: Clients should not scratch inside casts because of the risk of skin breakdown and potential damage to the cast. Option 4: Sedatives are not generally indicated for itching.

NP: Planning
CN: Physiological integrity
CNS: Reduction of risk potential
CL: Application

---

58 A 63-year-old man has a 10-year history of rheumatoid arthritis. He complains of stiff joints in the morning when he wakes up. On physical examination, you find that his knees are acutely inflamed. Which of the following would best help relieve the pain in his knees?

- ☐ 1. Increase physical activity such as walking.
- ☐ 2. Take two acetaminophen (Tylenol) tablets every 4 hours until the inflammation decreases.
- ☐ 3. Use ice packs on inflamed knees.
- ☐ 4. Use a heating pad continuously during the night.

CORRECT ANSWER: 3

Many clients with acute rheumatoid arthritis find some relief from cold application. Option 1: Physical activity during episodes of acute pain can prolong the crisis. Option 2: Acetaminophen has no anti-inflammatory action against rheumatoid arthritis. Option 4: Keeping a heating pad on through the night could burn the elderly client.

NP: Planning
CN: Physiological integrity
CNS: Physiological adaptation
CL: Application

59 A 26-year-old woman is admitted to the hospital after being involved in a motor vehicle accident. X-rays reveal that she has a comminuted fracture of the left femur. Which of the following best explains why narcotics are contraindicated for the leg pain?

☐ 1. She cannot provide a medical history.
☐ 2. She has diabetes with a high blood glucose count.
☐ 3. An open reduction of the fracture is anticipated.
☐ 4. A head injury is suspected and is being evaluated.

CORRECT ANSWER: 4
Narcotics are contraindicated in trauma cases because of the depressive effect on the respiratory center, which can result in hypoxia and increased ICP. Option 1: All medications would need to be given with caution if there is no medical history. Nothing specifically makes narcotics more contraindicated than other drugs. Option 2: Narcotics should be used with caution in diabetic clients, but they are not flatly contraindicated. Option 3: This situation in itself would not contraindicate narcotics.

NP: Planning
CN: Physiological integrity
CNS: Reduction of risk potential
CL: Application

---

60 A 65-year-old man comes to the ED with severe chest pain and shortness of breath. He is diaphoretic, pale, and weak. Suddenly, the client collapses and becomes unresponsive. What should the nurse do first when assessing an unresponsive client?

☐ 1. Check for a carotid pulse.
☐ 2. Check for spontaneous respirations.
☐ 3. Maintain an open airway.
☐ 4. Gently shake and shout, "Are you OK?"

CORRECT ANSWER: 4
Assessing level of consciousness (LOC) is the first step in basic life support. Unconsciousness is confirmed by shaking the client's shoulders and shouting, "Are you OK?" Option 1: Checking for circulation by palpating the carotid pulse is the fourth step. Options 2 and 3: The second step is to check for respirations and open the airway.

NP: Assessment
CN: Physiological integrity
CNS: Physiological adaptation
CL: Analysis

---

61 A client with heart failure develops pink frothy sputum, coarse crackles, and restlessness. Which of the following actions should the nurse take first?

☐ 1. Check the client's blood pressure.
☐ 2. Place the client in high Fowler's position.
☐ 3. Calculate the client's fluid balance.
☐ 4. Notify the physician.

CORRECT ANSWER: 2
Proper positioning can help reduce venous return to the heart. High Fowler's position also decreases lung congestion. Option 1 is important but does not take top priority. Option 3 would not be an immediate priority in an emergency. Option 4 should be done after the client has been repositioned and assessed.

NP: Implementation
CN: Physiological integrity
CNS: Physiological adaptation
CL: Analysis

62 While monitoring a client's cardiac rhythm, the nurse observes six multifocal premature ventricular contractions (PVCs) in a 1-minute strip. What action should the nurse take next?

- ☐ 1. Change electrocardiogram (ECG) leads.
- ☐ 2. Administer lidocaine (Xylocaine) per standing order.
- ☐ 3. Continue observation.
- ☐ 4. Ask the client to change position.

CORRECT ANSWER: 2

Multifocal PVCs occurring at six per minute increase the client's risk of ventricular fibrillation and should be treated. The most common agent used is lidocaine. Option 1: If the strip is clear, there is no problem with the leads. Options 3 and 4: Observation and position changes cannot suppress this potentially life-threatening arrhythmia.

NP: Implementation
CN: Physiological integrity
CNS: Physiological adaptation
CL: Application

---

63 A 74-year-old man with a history of heart failure is admitted to the coronary care unit with acute pulmonary edema. He is intubated and placed on a mechanical ventilator. Which of the following parameters should the nurse closely monitor in assessing the client's response to a bolus dose of I.V. furosemide (Lasix)?

- ☐ 1. Daily weight
- ☐ 2. 24-hour intake and output
- ☐ 3. Serum sodium levels
- ☐ 4. Hourly urine output

CORRECT ANSWER: 4

Furosemide administered by I.V. bolus takes effect almost immediately (within 5 minutes). Options 1, 2, and 3 would span repeated doses of furosemide and so would be less valuable in monitoring the client's initial reaction to the drug.

NP: Evaluation
CN: Physiological integrity
CNS: Pharmacological and parenteral therapies
CL: Application

---

64 A 48-year-old foreman at a local electric company comes to the hospital complaining of severe substernal chest pain radiating down his left arm. He is admitted to the coronary care unit with a diagnosis of myocardial infarction (MI). Which of the following nursing assessment activities is a priority on admission to coronary care?

- ☐ 1. Begin ECG monitoring.
- ☐ 2. Obtain information about family history of heart disease.
- ☐ 3. Auscultate lung fields.
- ☐ 4. Determine if the client smokes.

CORRECT ANSWER: 1

ECG monitoring should be started as soon as possible; life-threatening arrhythmias are the leading cause of death in the 1st hours after MI. Options 2 and 4: These are not immediate priorities in the acute phase of MI. Data may be obtained from family members later. Option 3: Lung fields are auscultated after oxygenation and pain control needs are met.

NP: Assessment
CN: Physiological integrity
CNS: Reduction of risk potential
CL: Application

65 A 56-year-old male has a blood pressure of 146/96 mm Hg. Upon hearing the reading, he exclaims, "My pressure has never been this high. Will I need to take medication to reduce it?" Which of the following is the best response by the nurse?

☐ 1. "Yes. Hypertension is prevalent among males; it's fortunate we caught this during your routine examination."
☐ 2. "We will need to reevaluate your blood pressure because your age places you at high risk for hypertension."
☐ 3. "A single elevated blood pressure does not confirm hypertension. You will need to have your blood pressure reassessed several times before a diagnosis can be made."
☐ 4. "You have no need to worry. Your pressure is probably elevated because you're in the doctor's office."

CORRECT ANSWER: 3

Hypertension is confirmed by three readings with systolic pressure of at least 140 mm Hg and diastolic pressure of at least 90 mm Hg. Option 1 is premature. Option 2 is not as specific as Option 3 and also is insensitive to the client's anxiety. Option 4 gives false reassurance; the client does need to have his blood pressure reevaluated.

NP: Planning
CN: Health promotion and maintenance
CNS: Prevention and early detection of disease
CL: Application

---

66 The nurse must plan care for a 28-year-old female admitted with a diagnosis of myasthenia gravis. Which of the following times would be most appropriate for procedures and care to be completed?

☐ 1. All at one time to provide a longer rest period
☐ 2. Before meals to stimulate her appetite
☐ 3. In the morning, with frequent rest periods
☐ 4. Before bedtime to promote rest

CORRECT ANSWER: 3

Myasthenia gravis is characterized by extreme muscle weakness, which generally worsens after effort and improves with rest. Option 1: Procedures should be spaced to allow for rest in between. Option 2: Procedures should be avoided before meals, or the client may be too exhausted to eat. Option 4: Procedures should be avoided at bedtime.

NP: Planning
CN: Physiological integrity
CNS: Reduction of risk potential
CL: Application

67 A 37-year-old teacher is admitted to the hospital with complaints of weakness, incoordination, dizziness, and loss of balance. The diagnosis is multiple sclerosis (MS). Which of the following signs and symptoms, discovered during the history and physical assessment, is typical of MS?

☐ 1. Diplopia, history of increased fatigue, and decreased or absent deep tendon reflexes
☐ 2. Flexor spasm, clonus, and negative Babinski's reflex
☐ 3. Blurred vision, intention tremor, and urinary hesitancy
☐ 4. Hyperactive abdominal reflexes and history of unsteady gait and episodic paresthesia in both legs

CORRECT ANSWER: 3
Optic neuritis, leading to blurred vision, is a common early sign of MS, as is intention tremor (tremor when performing an activity). Nerve damage can cause urinary hesitancy. Option 1: In MS, deep tendon reflexes are increased or hyperactive. Option 2: A positive Babinski's reflex is found in MS. Option 4: Abdominal reflexes are absent with MS.

NP: Assessment
CN: Physiological integrity
CNS: Physiological adaptation
CL: Application

---

68 A 72-year-old client has been admitted to the medical-surgical unit from the ED with a diagnosis of left-sided stroke in evolution. In transferring him from the stretcher to his bed, the nurse notices that the client's respirations have a snoring quality. Which nursing action would be the first priority at this time?

☐ 1. Place the client in Fowler's position, with the head of the bed at a 45-degree angle.
☐ 2. Assess the client's ability to communicate his needs.
☐ 3. Position the client on his side, with the head of the bed slightly elevated.
☐ 4. Place all items that the client may need to the left side of the bed.

CORRECT ANSWER: 3
Stroke in evolution refers to neurologic changes that continue for 24 to 48 hours. The snoring respirations indicate airway obstruction caused by the tongue falling backward; turning the client on his side will clear the obstruction. Option 1 is inappropriate. The client's right-sided weakness would not permit him to stay in Fowler's position. Options 2 and 4 are important but do not take top priority at this time.

NP: Implementation
CN: Physiological integrity
CNS: Reduction of risk potential
CL: Application

---

69 A client is being discharged after successful same-day cataract surgery. The nurse instructs the client about permitted activities and those to avoid. Which of the following activities is permitted?

☐ 1. Cooking
☐ 2. Driving
☐ 3. Vacuuming
☐ 4. Washing hair in the shower

CORRECT ANSWER: 1
Cooking will not cause increased IOP. Options 2 and 3: The client should avoid driving and vacuuming because they require forward flexion and rapid, jerky movements. Option 4: The client should not shower and must wash hair with the head tilted back to prevent soap and water from entering the eye, which would predispose the client to infection.

NP: Implementation
CN: Physiological integrity
CNS: Reduction of risk potential
CL: Application

70 About 4 hours after a client with cerebrovascular accident (CVA) is admitted, the nurse obtains these vital signs: blood pressure, 170/80 mm Hg; apical pulse, 58 beats/minute with a regular rhythm; respiratory rate, 14 breaths/minute; axillary temperature, 101 °F (38.3 °C). Which nursing action at this time is most appropriate?

- ☐ 1. Call the physician to report the vital signs.
- ☐ 2. Assess vital signs more frequently.
- ☐ 3. Assess the client for an overdistended bladder.
- ☐ 4. Assess the client for signs of overhydration.

CORRECT ANSWER: 1

Brain injury can either elevate or depress blood pressure. A slow pulse, decreased respiratory rate, and increased pulse pressure also are associated with CVA. Option 2: Although the frequency of assessment will no doubt be increased, the top priority is to report the client's vital signs to the physician. Option 3: The listed vital signs are associated with increased ICP and do not result from a distended bladder. Option 4: The vital signs are not associated with fluid overload.

NP: Implementation
CN: Physiological integrity
CNS: Physiological adaptation
CL: Analysis

---

71 A client who has sustained a head injury is to receive mannitol (Osmitrol) by I.V. push. In evaluating the effectiveness of the drug, the nurse should expect to find which of the following?

- ☐ 1. Increased lung expansion
- ☐ 2. Decreased cerebral edema
- ☐ 3. Decreased cardiac workload
- ☐ 4. Increased cerebral circulation

CORRECT ANSWER: 2

Mannitol, an osmotic diuretic, is used to decrease cerebral edema in clients with head injuries. Options 1, 3, and 4 are not effects of mannitol.

NP: Evaluation
CN: Physiological integrity
CNS: Pharmacological and parenteral therapies
CL: Application

---

72 An ambulatory client has just returned from the X-ray department, where a cervical myelogram with a water-based dye was performed. Which of the following actions should postprocedure nursing care include?

- ☐ 1. Force fluids.
- ☐ 2. Maintain the client flat in bed for 12 hours.
- ☐ 3. Turn the client from side to side after 2 hours.
- ☐ 4. Monitor blood glucose for 24 hours.

CORRECT ANSWER: 1

After having a myelogram with a water-based dye, the client is encouraged to drink liberal amounts of fluid for rehydration and replacement of cerebrospinal fluid (CSF). Option 2: The client should be positioned with the head of the bed elevated to pool the dye at the lower end of the spinal canal; this will help prevent irritation of the meninges. Option 3: Bathroom privileges are granted, but unnecessary turning is not advised for the first few hours. Option 4: Blood glucose monitoring is not essential.

NP: Implementation
CN: Physiological integrity
CNS: Reduction of risk potential
CL: Application

73 A client with a neurogenic bladder is beginning bladder training. Which of the following nursing actions is most important?

☐ 1. Set up specific times to empty the bladder.
☐ 2. Force fluids.
☐ 3. Provide adequate roughage.
☐ 4. Encourage the use of an indwelling urinary catheter.

CORRECT ANSWER: 1

Clients are taught to write down their voiding pattern and to empty the bladder at the same times each day. Option 2: Forcing fluids (more than 2 L/day) increases urine production and complicates the initial bladder-training process. Option 3: Roughage is unnecessary for bladder training. Option 4: An indwelling urinary catheter is used only when other methods of control do not work.

NP: Planning
CN: Physiological integrity
CNS: Basic care and comfort
CL: Application

---

74 A client in the ED with a decreased LOC and symptoms of spinal shock begins to lose consciousness altogether. Blood pressure drops to 40/20 mm Hg. Shortly thereafter, the nurse notes ventricular tachycardia on the client's bedside monitor. Which of the following actions should the nurse take next?

☐ 1. Call for assistance from the physician and other nurses and await further orders.
☐ 2. Call for assistance and begin cardiopulmonary resuscitation (CPR).
☐ 3. Call for assistance and prepare to defibrillate the client, providing CPR until a defibrillator is available.
☐ 4. Administer 1 mg of atropine and begin CPR.

CORRECT ANSWER: 3

Clients in unstable ventricular tachycardia should always be defibrillated before other resuscitation efforts are instituted. If a defibrillator is not readily available, CPR should be started. Option 1: The nurse needs to act quickly and cannot await further orders. Option 2: Defibrillation should be done first. Option 4: Atropine administration would not be appropriate.

NP: Implementation
CN: Physiological integrity
CNS: Physiological adaptation
CL: Analysis

---

75 A 64-year-old female is found on the floor of her apartment. She had apparently fallen and hit her head on the bathtub. On admission to the neurologic unit, she has a decreased LOC. The physician orders positioning as follows: elevate the head of the bed; keep the head in neutral alignment with no neck flexion or head rotation; avoid sharp hip flexion. Which of the following is the best rationale for this positioning?

☐ 1. To decrease cerebral arterial pressure
☐ 2. To avoid impeding venous outflow
☐ 3. To prevent flexion contractures
☐ 4. To prevent aspiration of stomach contents

CORRECT ANSWER: 2

Any activity or position that impedes venous outflow from the head may contribute to increased volume inside the skull and possibly increase ICP. Option 1: Cerebral arterial pressure will be affected by the balance between oxygen and carbon dioxide. Option 3: Flexion contractures are not a priority at this time. Option 4: Stomach contents could still be aspirated in this position.

NP: Implementation
CN: Physiological integrity
CNS: Reduction of risk potential
CL: Application

76 A male client has a 10-year history of rheumatoid arthritis. For the past several weeks he has been taking 650 mg of aspirin every 4 hours. Which of the following would be most important for the nurse to teach him?

☐ 1. He is taking too much aspirin; he should stop taking it and consult his physician.
☐ 2. Any stomach complaints should be reported to his health care provider.
☐ 3. Easy bruising is a normal reaction that he can expect from the aspirin therapy.
☐ 4. He will get better pain relief from lower doses of aspirin if he takes it between meals.

CORRECT ANSWER: 2

GI distress is a common adverse effect of aspirin and can result in GI bleeding. Option 1: This amount of aspirin is typical for rheumatoid arthritis clients. Option 3: Bruising, which indicates prolonged bleeding, must be reported. Option 4: Aspirin causes fewer GI complaints if taken with food.

NP: Implementation
CN: Physiological integrity
CNS: Pharmacological and parenteral therapies
CL: Application

---

77 A 58-year-old male is admitted for a wedge resection of the left lower lung lobe. A routine chest X-ray shows carcinoma. The client is anxious and asks if he can smoke. Which of the following statements by the nurse would be most therapeutic?

☐ 1. "Smoking is the reason you are here."
☐ 2. "The doctor left orders for you not to smoke."
☐ 3. "You're anxious about the surgery. Do you see smoking as helping?"
☐ 4. "Smoking now is OK, but after your surgery it's contraindicated."

CORRECT ANSWER: 3

This acknowledges the client's feelings and encourages him to assess his previous behavior. Option 1 belittles the client. Option 2 does not address the client's anxiety. Option 4 would be highly detrimental to this client.

NP: Implementation
CN: Psychosocial integrity
CNS: Coping and adaptation
CL: Application

---

78 A female client is discharged from the hospital after having an episode of heart failure. She is prescribed daily oral doses of digoxin (Lanoxin) and furosemide (Lasix). Two days later, she tells her community health nurse that she feels weak and frequently feels her heart "flutter." What would be the nurse's best action?

☐ 1. Tell the client to rest more often.
☐ 2. Tell the client to stop taking the digoxin, and call the physician.
☐ 3. Call the physician, report the symptoms, and request to draw a blood sample to determine the client's potassium level.
☐ 4. Tell the client to avoid foods that contain caffeine.

CORRECT ANSWER: 3

Furosemide is a potassium-wasting diuretic. A low potassium level may cause weakness and palpitations. Option 1: This will not help the client if she is hypokalemic. Option 2: The digoxin is not causing the client's symptoms. Option 4: The client should probably avoid caffeine, but this would not resolve potassium depletion.

NP: Implementation
CN: Physiological integrity
CNS: Pharmacological and parenteral therapies
CL: Application

79 A male client with a total hip replacement is progressing well and expects to be discharged tomorrow. On returning to bed after ambulating, he complains of severe pain in the surgical wound. Which action should the nurse take?

☐ 1. Assume he is anxious about discharge, and administer pain medication.
☐ 2. Assess the surgical site and affected extremity.
☐ 3. Reassure the client that pain is a direct result of increased activity.
☐ 4. Suspect a wound infection, and monitor the client's temperature and vital signs.

CORRECT ANSWER: 2

Worsening pain after a total hip replacement may indicate dislocation of the prosthesis. Assessment of pain should include evaluation of the wound and the affected extremity. Option 1: This does not address the cause of the pain. Option 3: Sudden severe pain is not normal after hip replacement. Option 4: Wound infections are usually distinguished by purulent drainage.

NP: Assessment
CN: Physiological integrity
CNS: Physiological adaptation
CL: Analysis

---

80 A client sustains a C5 spinal cord injury that results in quadriplegia. Several days after being moved out of the intensive care unit, he complains of a severe throbbing headache. What should the nurse do next?

☐ 1. Check the client's indwelling urinary catheter for kinks to ensure patency.
☐ 2. Lower the head of the bed to improve perfusion.
☐ 3. Call the physician immediately for a pain medication order.
☐ 4. Reassure the client that headaches are normal after spinal cord injuries.

CORRECT ANSWER: 1

A severe throbbing headache is a common symptom of autonomic dysreflexia, which occurs after injuries to the spinal cord above T6. The syndrome is usually brought on by sympathetic stimulation, such as bowel and bladder distention. Option 2: Lowering the head of the bed can increase ICP. Option 3: Before calling the physician, the nurse should check the client's catheter, record vital signs, and perform an abdominal assessment. Option 4: A severe throbbing headache is a dangerous symptom in this client; it is not normal.

NP: Implementation
CN: Physiological integrity
CNS: Physiological adaptation
CL: Analysis

81 A male client, age 55, has been diagnosed with open-angle glaucoma. The physician's orders include one drop of pilocarpine hydrochloride (Pilocar) 1% in each eye, every 6 hours. The client states that he doesn't understand the need for medication because he doesn't have symptoms of an eye problem. Which of the following nursing diagnoses would be most appropriate?

- ☐ 1. Noncompliance related to refusal to use eyedrops
- ☐ 2. Risk for altered health maintenance related to insufficient knowledge of the disease
- ☐ 3. Anxiety related to a new health problem
- ☐ 4. Body image disturbance related to the need for medication

Correct answer: 2

Risk for altered health maintenance is the nursing diagnosis used for an individual who lacks the knowledge to manage a condition. Option 1: Noncompliance does not apply to clients who refuse treatment but to those who fail to follow an agreed-upon treatment plan. Options 3 and 4: Assessment data do not support these diagnoses.

NP: Planning
CN: Physiological integrity
CNS: Reduction of risk potential
CL: Application

---

82 A 42-year-old male has been diagnosed with tuberculosis (TB). He is concerned about when he can return to his job as a department store manager because he has a large family to support. Which of the following statements would be the best basis for the nurse's response?

- ☐ 1. Clients with TB must complete chemotherapy treatments before they are considered noncontagious.
- ☐ 2. Clients with TB may resume normal activities after hospitalization; however, they must wear masks when in contact with nonfamily members.
- ☐ 3. Clients with TB usually are not restricted in their activities for more than 4 weeks after chemotherapy is begun, provided that they comply with the medication regimen.
- ☐ 4. Clients with TB are always considered contagious and must have limitations placed on them for life.

Correct answer: 3

Clients who comply with the medication regimen are not considered contagious after hospitalization. Barring complications, they may resume normal activities. Options 1 and 4: Although the course of treatment may take longer than 9 months, clients are considered noncontagious when they have produced three consecutive sputum specimens free from *Mycobacterium tuberculosis* (usually within 2 weeks after beginning chemotherapy). Option 2: Clients with TB should continue to cover their mouths with tissues when coughing; however, masks are not routinely worn after hospitalization.

NP: Planning
CN: Physiological integrity
CNS: Pharmacological and parenteral therapies
CL: Application

83 A client with a positive Mantoux test is taking isoniazid (INH) as prescribed. Which of the following should the nurse assess for during the client's next clinic visit?

☐ 1. Right upper quadrant abdominal pain
☐ 2. Peripheral edema
☐ 3. Shortness of breath
☐ 4. Pruritus

CORRECT ANSWER: 1

The nurse should assess for signs of liver dysfunction because up to 20% of clients taking isoniazid show signs of hepatic stress. Option 2: Peripheral edema is associated with heart failure. Options 3 and 4: Neither shortness of breath nor pruritus is typically associated with isoniazid administration.

NP: Assessment
CN: Physiological integrity
CNS: Pharmacological and parenteral therapies
CL: Application

---

84 Which nursing action takes priority when admitting a client with right lower lobe pneumonia?

☐ 1. Elevate the head of the bed 45 to 90 degrees.
☐ 2. Auscultate the chest for adventitious sounds.
☐ 3. Obtain a sputum specimen for culture.
☐ 4. Notify the physician of the client's admission.

CORRECT ANSWER: 1

Clients with pneumonia will breathe easier in Fowler's or semi-Fowler's position because gravity facilitates diaphragmatic movement. Options 2, 3, and 4 are important but do not have first priority.

NP: Implementation
CN: Physiological integrity
CNS: Reduction of risk potential
CL: Application

---

85 A male client has had a segmental left lung resection for treatment of a lung carcinoma. He returns from surgery with a left posterior-lateral chest tube attached to a disposable water-seal chest drainage system. Which of the following would indicate that the drainage system is working properly?

☐ 1. Air is bubbling in the water-seal chamber.
☐ 2. The fluid level in the drainage chamber remains constant.
☐ 3. The fluid level in the water-seal chamber fluctuates.
☐ 4. A pneumothorax is present.

CORRECT ANSWER: 3

Fluctuation of the fluid level (upward on inspiration and downward on exhalation) in the water-seal chamber indicates a patent tube. Option 1: Bubbling in the water-seal chamber indicates an air leak. Option 2: A constant fluid level in the drainage chamber may indicate an obstructed drainage tube. Option 4: A pneumothorax would not indicate whether the drainage equipment was functioning properly.

NP: Assessment
CN: Physiological integrity
CNS: Reduction of risk potential
CL: Analysis

86 A 57-year-old client is admitted to the hospital for exacerbation of COPD. Which of the following would the nurse expect to find during a nursing assessment?

☐ 1. Dyspnea, cough, and bradycardia
☐ 2. Wheezing, tachycardia, and restlessness
☐ 3. Barrel chest, tachycardia, and hypertension
☐ 4. Hypotension, confusion, and weight gain

CORRECT ANSWER: 2

Wheezing results when air is expired against a collapsed airway; tachycardia results from hypoxia; and restlessness results from cerebral hypoxia. Option 1: Bradycardia is not present in COPD. Option 3: Hypertension is not present in COPD. Option 4: Many clients with COPD experience anorexia and subsequent weight loss, not weight gain.

NP: Assessment
CN: Physiological integrity
CNS: Physiological adaptation
CL: Analysis

---

87 The nurse is assessing a client for signs of hypoxemia. Which of the following should the nurse interpret as a late sign of hypoxemia?

☐ 1. Increased respiratory rate
☐ 2. Increased heart rate
☐ 3. Diaphoresis
☐ 4. Agitation

CORRECT ANSWER: 3

Initially, the respiratory rate increases to obtain more oxygen, the heart rate increases in response to increased energy demands, and the client experiences agitation from early cerebral hypoxia. Later, as the client continues to work to obtain oxygen, the skin becomes diaphoretic and cool from vasoconstriction. Options 1, 2, and 4 are early signs of hypoxemia.

NP: Assessment
CN: Physiological integrity
CNS: Physiological adaptation
CL: Analysis

---

88 A client with a hyperactive goiter is alert and oriented but anxious, with fine hand tremors and rapid speech. Which of the following rooms would be best for the client?

☐ 1. One with a temperature between 65°and 68°F (18.3°and 20°C)
☐ 2. One near the nurses' station
☐ 3. One with a temperature between 75°F and 78°F (23.9°and 25.6°C)
☐ 4. One with a private bathroom

CORRECT ANSWER: 1

The client's symptoms indicate hyperthyroidism. Clients with hyperthyroidism have heat intolerance and need a room cooler than the average. Option 2: Clients with hyperthyroidism need an environment with decreased stimulation. A room near the nurses' station does not meet this requirement. Option 3: This environment would be too warm for a client with hyperthyroidism. Option 4: A private bathroom may be a desirable amenity, but it is more important to have a room with a suitable temperature.

NP: Planning
CN: Physiological integrity
CNS: Physiological adaptation
CL: Application

89 A 26-year-old male client is in the ED after a motorcycle accident. His blood pressure falls to 70/50 mm Hg, his pulse slows to 50 beats/minute, and he cannot move his legs. Which of the following actions should the nurse take next?

☐ 1. Open the clamp on the client's I.V. line to speed the flow rate of fluid.
☐ 2. Leave the room to find the physician immediately.
☐ 3. Remain with the client and ask another nurse to locate the physician immediately.
☐ 4. Administer 1 mg of epinephrine to maintain the client's blood pressure.

CORRECT ANSWER: 3

A client experiencing spinal shock with hypotension and neurologic changes should not be left alone, and the physician must be summoned. Option 1: Giving additional I.V. fluid may be contraindicated because of the potential for cerebral edema. Option 2: The client should not be left alone. Option 4: Other orders should be obtained from the physician to maintain blood pressure; administration of epinephrine is not appropriate for treatment of hypotension caused by spinal shock.

NP: Implementation
CN: Physiological integrity
CNS: Physiological adaptation
CL: Analysis

---

90 A client with hyperthyroidism is started on propylthiouracil. When should the nurse expect noticeable improvement in the client's condition?

☐ 1. In 24 to 48 hours
☐ 2. In 6 to 7 days
☐ 3. In 2 to 4 weeks
☐ 4. In 6 months

CORRECT ANSWER: 3

Propylthiouracil is slow-acting, taking 2 to 4 weeks to produce noticeable improvement. Options 1, 2, and 4 are incorrect.

NP: Evaluation
CN: Physiological integrity
CNS: Pharmacological and parenteral therapies
CL: Application

---

91 A client is to begin taking vasopressin (Pitressin). Which of the following statements would indicate proper understanding of client teaching?

☐ 1. "I will increase my daily dosage of vasopressin if I experience headaches or abdominal cramps."
☐ 2. "I will drink a full glass of water with each oral dose of vasopressin."
☐ 3. "I should shake the ampule of medicine thoroughly before drawing the dose for administration."
☐ 4. "I should have increased urine output as a result of taking this drug."

CORRECT ANSWER: 3

Ampules of vasopressin should be shaken thoroughly to dissolve the solute before drug administration. Option 1: Vasopressin can cause headaches and abdominal cramps. If these occur, the physician may decrease the dosage. Option 2: Vasopressin is administered parenterally. If given orally, it would be destroyed by enzyme activity in the stomach. Option 4: The client can expect reduced urine output for 24 to 96 hours after taking vasopressin.

NP: Evaluation
CN: Physiological integrity
CNS: Pharmacological and parenteral therapies
CL: Analysis

92 A male client, age 78, has been newly diagnosed with hypothyroidism. He lives in his own apartment in a community development designed for the elderly. He asks the nurse assigned to this complex for advice about his condition. What would be the best advice the nurse could give the client?

- ☐ 1. "Stop taking your self-prescribed daily aspirin."
- ☐ 2. "Stop attending group activities."
- ☐ 3. "Keep the temperature in your apartment cooler than usual."
- ☐ 4. "Increase fiber and fluids in your diet."

CORRECT ANSWER: 4

Clients with hypothyroidism typically have constipation. A diet high in fiber and fluids can help prevent this. Option 1: Taking aspirin is not related to hypothyroidism management. Option 2: The client does not need to discontinue all group activities, although he may need to limit them until his condition improves. Option 3: Clients with hypothyroidism have an intolerance to cold and need an environment warmer than average.

NP: Implementation
CN: Physiological integrity
CNS: Physiological adaptation
CL: Application

---

93 A 28-year-old female has had type 1 diabetes for 10 years. She is doing home glucose monitoring and urinary dipsticks for acetone. She asks the nurse why she has to dipstick her urine, too. Which of the following rationales should the nurse use in response?

- ☐ 1. A positive test reaction indicates too much glucose.
- ☐ 2. A positive test reaction indicates too much insulin.
- ☐ 3. A positive test reaction indicates ketoacidosis.
- ☐ 4. The test measures protein in the urine.

CORRECT ANSWER: 3

Urinary acetone indicates the development of ketoacidosis from the body's breakdown of fats. Option 1: The test does not measure glucose; rather, it measures ketone bodies that are formed when fats are being metabolized for energy. Options 2 and 4: The test does not measure either insulin or protein.

NP: Implementation
CN: Physiological integrity
CNS: Reduction of risk potential
CL: Application

---

94 A 45-year-old chemistry teacher is recovering from a left pneumonectomy necessitated by lung cancer. Which of the following postoperative positions would be best for this client?

- ☐ 1. Prone or on the operative side, with the head elevated
- ☐ 2. Prone or on the unaffected side, with the head elevated
- ☐ 3. Supine or on the operative side, with the head elevated
- ☐ 4. Supine or on the unaffected side, with the head elevated

CORRECT ANSWER: 3

After a pneumonectomy, closed chest drainage is generally not used. For optimal expansion of the remaining lung, lying supine or on the operative side is recommended. Options 1 and 2: The prone position is not appropriate. Option 4: Lying on the unaffected side will impair ventilation of the remaining lung.

NP: Implementation
CN: Physiological integrity
CNS: Reduction of risk potential
CL: Application

95 The nurse is teaching a client about the adverse effects of tamoxifen (Nolvadex). Which of the following adverse effects should the nurse teach the client to report?

☐ 1. Vaginal bleeding, hot flashes, and weight gain
☐ 2. Increased libido, acne, and facial hirsutism
☐ 3. Mouth sores, diarrhea, and appetite loss
☐ 4. Increased blood pressure, insomnia, and mood swings

CORRECT ANSWER: 1

Vaginal bleeding, hot flashes, and weight gain are common adverse effects of tamoxifen. Option 2: These adverse effects are associated with androgen therapy. Option 3: These signs and symptoms are associated with chemotherapy. Option 4: These adverse effects are associated with corticosteroids.

NP: Implementation
CN: Physiological integrity
CNS: Pharmacological and parenteral therapies
CL: Application

---

96 A client is scheduled for a cholecystectomy. After the nurse completes the preoperative teaching, the client states, "If I lie still and avoid turning, I will avoid pain. Do you think this is a good idea?" What is the nurse's best response?

☐ 1. "It is always a good idea to rest quietly after surgery."
☐ 2. "You need to turn from side to side every 2 hours."
☐ 3. "The doctor will probably order you to lie flat for 24 hours."
☐ 4. "Why don't you decide about activity after you return from the recovery room?"

CORRECT ANSWER: 2

To prevent venous stasis and to improve muscle tone, circulation, and respiratory function, the client should be encouraged to move about after surgery. Pain medication will be administered to permit movement. Options 1 and 3: The client must turn and ambulate to prevent atelectasis. Option 4: Activity should not be left entirely to the client's discretion.

NP: Evaluation
CN: Physiological integrity
CNS: Reduction of risk potential
CL: Application

---

97 A 46-year-old male has come to the ED for treatment for chest pain. After the pain subsides, he is admitted to a medical-surgical unit with telemetry because no cardiac unit beds are available. In reviewing the client's laboratory results 6 hours later, the nurse notices that his creatine kinase isoenzymes (CK-MB) are markedly elevated. What action should the nurse take next?

☐ 1. None; this is expected with all anginal episodes.
☐ 2. Ask for another blood sample; a laboratory error is likely.
☐ 3. Notify the physician and prepare the client for transfer to the cardiac care unit.
☐ 4. Infuse I.V. potassium to protect against arrhythmias.

CORRECT ANSWER: 3

CK levels rise within 4 to 8 hours after myocardial injury. The amount of increase usually corresponds to the size of the infarct. Option 1: Elevated CK levels are not expected after angina; rather, they indicate cell death that occurs after an infarct. Option 2: No data exist to suspect laboratory error. Option 4: This would be an inappropriate nursing action.

NP: Implementation
CN: Physiological integrity
CNS: Reduction of risk potential
CL: Analysis

98 An 81-year-old man is admitted to the hospital with a diagnosis of streptococcal pneumonia. Which finding would the nurse expect while doing a physical assessment?

☐ 1. History of gradual onset of illness, tachypnea, and fever
☐ 2. Shortness of breath, bradycardia, and fever
☐ 3. Chest pain, tachycardia, and headache
☐ 4. Cough, crackles, and bradypnea

CORRECT ANSWER: 3

Chest pain and headache commonly occur with streptococcal pneumonia. Tachycardia results from hypoxia. Option 1: Streptococcal pneumonia usually has a sudden onset. Option 2: Clients with pneumonia usually have tachycardia, not bradycardia. Option 4: Clients with pneumonia usually have tachypnea, not bradypnea.

NP: Assessment
CN: Physiological integrity
CNS: Physiological adaptation
CL: Application

---

99 A client with COPD is being discharged after treatment for an acute exacerbation. Which statement by the client indicates proper understanding of the discharge instructions?

☐ 1. "I should take my bronchodilator at bedtime to prevent insomnia."
☐ 2. "I should do my most difficult activities when I first get up in the morning."
☐ 3. "I should try to eat several small meals during the day."
☐ 4. "I should plan to do my exercises after I eat."

CORRECT ANSWER: 3

Because digestion takes energy that they need to devote to breathing instead, COPD clients may feel full after only a small meal. They may better tolerate smaller, more frequent high-calorie meals. Option 1: Bronchodilators may contribute to insomnia. Option 2: Most COPD clients tolerate activity better if it is spaced throughout the day, with frequent rest periods. Option 4: A client participating in an exercise rehabilitation program should exercise before eating.

NP: Evaluation
CN: Physiological integrity
CNS: Basic care and comfort
CL: Analysis

---

100 A client has been admitted after suffering a CVA. Some 24 hours after admission, the client has right-sided hemiplegia. Which of the following neurologic deficits is closely associated with this type of hemiplegia?

☐ 1. Difficulty speaking and understanding
☐ 2. Loss of consciousness
☐ 3. Inability to see to the left
☐ 4. Poor judgment and impulsive behavior

CORRECT ANSWER: 1

Right-sided hemiplegia is caused by damage to the left hemisphere of the brain. Expressive and receptive dysphasias are associated with damage to the left hemisphere, where the dominant speech centers are located in most people. Option 2: Loss of consciousness can result from any type of CVA. Option 3: A client with left-hemisphere damage will more likely have difficulty with vision on the right side. Option 4: Poor judgment and impulsive behavior are associated with damage to the right hemisphere.

NP: Evaluation
CN: Physiological integrity
CNS: Physiological adaptation
CL: Application

101 A 32-year-old client with epilepsy is admitted for treatment of an acute asthma attack. A history reveals that theophylline (Theo-Dur) has been prescribed. Which of the following might indicate that the client has not been taking the medication as prescribed?

- ☐ 1. The client complains of nervousness, headache, and palpitations.
- ☐ 2. The nurse hears sneezes as she auscultates the chest.
- ☐ 3. The client's blood theophylline level is 5 mg/ml.
- ☐ 4. The client has had increased episodes of seizure activity.

CORRECT ANSWER: 3
A therapeutic serum theophylline level is 10 to 20 mg/ml. A level lower than 10 mg/ml indicates that the client has not been receiving a therapeutic dose. Option 1: Nervousness, palpitations, and headache are common adverse effects of theophylline. Option 2: Sneezing does not indicate noncompliance. Option 4: Seizure activity is a potential adverse effect of theophylline therapy.

NP: Evaluation
CN: Physiological integrity
CNS: Pharmacological and parenteral therapies
CL: Application

---

102 A client comes to the clinic because of low-grade afternoon fevers, night sweats, and a productive cough. The physician suspects pulmonary tuberculosis, especially after the client remarks that his wife was recently diagnosed with the disease. A positive acid-fast bacillus sputum culture confirms the diagnosis of tuberculosis. During an initial nursing history, you observe that the client refers to his diagnosis by using the impersonal pronoun "it." What would be your best response?

- ☐ 1. "Let's not talk about it. How long have you been having night sweats?"
- ☐ 2. "Tell me how you feel about the diagnosis of tuberculosis."
- ☐ 3. "'It' will not kill you if you take your medications."
- ☐ 4. "You should not be embarrassed that you have tuberculosis."

CORRECT ANSWER: 2
This allows the client to express his feelings about the diagnosis. Option 1 ignores the client's feelings. Option 3 belittles the client. Option 4 is presumptive and judgmental.

NP: Assessment
CN: Psychosocial integrity
CNS: Coping and adaptation
CL: Analysis

---

103 A client's arterial blood gas (ABG) analysis reveals a carbon dioxide excess. The nurse should recognize that this is consistent with which one of the following?

- ☐ 1. Metabolic acidosis
- ☐ 2. Metabolic alkalosis
- ☐ 3. Respiratory acidosis
- ☐ 4. Respiratory alkalosis

CORRECT ANSWER: 3
An increased level of dissolved carbon dioxide ($Paco_2$) indicates respiratory acidosis. Option 1: Metabolic acidosis is indicated by a decreased bicarbonate (HCO_3-) level. Option 2: Metabolic alkalosis is an excess of HCO_3-. Option 4: Respiratory alkalosis is indicated by a decreased $Paco_2$ level.

NP: Evaluation
CN: Physiological integrity
CNS: Physiological adaptation
CL: Analysis

104 A nurse is preparing to teach a client about the effects of isoniazid (INH). Which of the following must the nurse be sure that the client understands?

- ☐ 1. Drinking alcohol daily can increase the incidence of drug-induced hepatitis.
- ☐ 2. Taking aluminum hydroxide (Maalox) with isoniazid minimizes GI upset.
- ☐ 3. The medication is absorbed best when taken on an empty stomach.
- ☐ 4. Prolonged use of isoniazid produces poorly concentrated urine.

CORRECT ANSWER: 1
Drinking alcohol can induce isoniazid-related hepatitis. Option 2: Clients should avoid concomitant use of aluminum-containing antacids with isoniazid. Option 3: Isoniazid taken with meals decreases GI upset. Option 4: If hepatic damage occurs, the client's urine may become dark and appear concentrated.

NP: Planning
CN: Physiological integrity
CNS: Pharmacological and parenteral therapies
CL: Application

---

105 A client with COPD and worsening dyspnea continues to deteriorate and needs a more accurate method for oxygen delivery. Which of the following oxygen delivery systems is the best to use?

- ☐ 1. Nasal prongs
- ☐ 2. Simple face mask
- ☐ 3. Nonrebreathing mask
- ☐ 4. Venturi mask

CORRECT ANSWER: 4
The Venturi mask delivers the most accurate concentrations of oxygen. An adapter located between the bottom of the mask and the oxygen inlet regulates the mixture of pure oxygen and atmospheric air to deliver the exact percentage of oxygen stipulated by the set flow rate. Options 1, 2, and 3: None of these methods delivers oxygen as precisely as the Venturi mask.

NP: Implementation
CN: Physiological integrity
CNS: Physiological adaptation
CL: Application

---

106 The primary antitubercular drug isoniazid (INH) is prescribed for a client, along with pyridoxine hydrochloride (vitamin B_6). What is the purpose of pyridoxine?

- ☐ 1. To enhance the action of isoniazid
- ☐ 2. To prevent the adverse effects of isoniazid on the central nervous system
- ☐ 3. To aid in the absorption of isoniazid from the stomach
- ☐ 4. To stimulate the maturation of red blood cells

CORRECT ANSWER: 2
Pyridoxine can be used to prevent the development of peripheral neuropathy in clients taking isoniazid. Options 1, 3, and 4: These are not actions of pyridoxine.

NP: Implementation
CN: Physiological integrity
CNS: Pharmacological and parenteral therapies
CL: Comprehension

107 A client is scheduled for an EEG. Which of the following would the client be permitted to ingest during the 24 hours before the test?

☐ 1. Coffee and tea
☐ 2. Solid foods
☐ 3. Stimulants
☐ 4. Tranquilizers

CORRECT ANSWER: 2

Solid foods are permitted. Options 1, 3, and 4: Stimulants, including the caffeine in coffee and tea, and tranquilizers can alter EEG wave patterns or mask abnormal patterns. Therefore, such substances must be avoided for 24 hours before the test.

NP: Implementation
CN: Physiological integrity
CNS: Reduction of risk potential
CL: Application

---

108 A female client with MS was admitted to the hospital with symptoms of visual impairment. The symptoms have resolved, and the client is being discharged. She asks if she can continue her twice-weekly workouts at exercise class. Which of the following is the best response by the nurse?

☐ 1. "Even moderate exercise can contribute to the recurrence of your symptoms."
☐ 2. "Prolonged exercise increases muscle strength and endurance."
☐ 3. "Active exercise is helpful in relieving muscle spasticity."
☐ 4. "It is important to exercise, but you should stop short of fatigue."

CORRECT ANSWER: 4

Exercise is essential to strengthen weak muscles during periods of remission, but vigorous exercise to the point of fatigue may aggravate symptoms. Option 1: Moderate exercise is beneficial. Option 2: Prolonged exercise is not recommended. Option 3: Exercise will not relieve spasticity.

NP: Implementation
CN: Health promotion and maintenance
CNS: Prevention and early detection of disease
CL: Application

---

109 A client had a segmental lung resection 3 days ago, and a chest X-ray confirms that the lung has reexpanded. The surgeon is preparing to remove the chest tube. What should the nurse instruct the client to do during chest tube removal?

☐ 1. Inhale deeply.
☐ 2. Exhale deeply.
☐ 3. Cough intermittently.
☐ 4. Breathe normally.

CORRECT ANSWER: 2

The goal is to prevent air from entering the pleural cavity as the tube is withdrawn. Options 1 and 4: These would allow air to enter the pleural cavity during chest tube removal. Option 3: Coughing causes jarring and interferes with tube removal.

NP: Implementation
CN: Physiological integrity
CNS: Reduction of risk potential
CL: Application

110 An elderly male client is admitted with a diagnosis of bacterial pneumonia. He is experiencing moderate dyspnea, a fever of 102°F (38.9°C), fatigue, and chest pain on inspiration. He complains of shortness of breath, and his respiratory rate increases to 36 breaths/minute after eating breakfast and having his morning care. What would be the best plan for the nurse to implement?

☐ 1. Continue the same plan of care.
☐ 2. Help the client with his breakfast, and omit morning care.
☐ 3. Plan for a rest period between breakfast and morning care.
☐ 4. Have the client cough and deep-breathe after breakfast, and then give morning care.

CORRECT ANSWER: 3
Planning rest periods between activities will increase the client's tolerance for activity and should reduce his shortness of breath, allowing him to maintain something closer to a normal respiratory rate. Option 1 will not decrease his activity or ease his metabolic demand. Option 2 makes the client dependent and does not address his hygiene needs. Option 4 increases the client's activity and energy demands.

NP: Planning
CN: Physiological integrity
CNS: Basic care and comfort
CL: Application

---

111 A client who has suffered a closed head injury has been placed on a cooling blanket and given an antipyretic, as prescribed. In evaluating the client's response to these treatments, the nurse should anticipate that the therapeutic effects of these measures will do which of the following?

☐ 1. Prevent hypoxia secondary to diaphoresis
☐ 2. Promote integrity of intracerebral neurons
☐ 3. Promote equalization of osmotic factors
☐ 4. Reduce brain metabolism and limit brain hypoxia

CORRECT ANSWER: 4
ICP increases with hyperpyrexia. Hypothermia, which may be achieved with cooling blankets and antipyretics, reduces brain metabolism and makes it less vulnerable to hypoxia. Option 1: Diaphoresis is merely a sign of increased temperature or decreased cardiac output. Options 2 and 3: These depend on an adequate supply of oxygen, carbon dioxide, hydrogen ions, glucose, and other factors.

NP: Evaluation
CN: Physiological integrity
CNS: Physiological adaptation
CL: Application

---

112 The physician orders ABG analysis to be done 12 hours after removing a chest tube from a client. Analysis reveals that the client's partial pressure of arterial oxygen (Pao_2) value is 90 mm Hg. What should the nurse do next?

☐ 1. Provide oxygen supplementation.
☐ 2. Have the client cough and deep-breathe every 2 hours.
☐ 3. Notify the physician of the ABG results.
☐ 4. Take no action; the client's Pao_2 is adequate.

CORRECT ANSWER: 4
The normal Pao_2 value is 80 to 95 mm Hg. Options 1, 2, and 3 are unnecessary.

NP: Evaluation
CN: Physiological integrity
CNS: Physiological adaptation
CL: Analysis

113 In assessing the cardiopulmonary system of a client with heart failure, the nurse identifies a third heart sound (S_3) on auscultation. What is the most likely significance of this finding?

☐ 1. Incomplete closing of the semilunar valves
☐ 2. Normal cardiac physiology
☐ 3. Atrial incompetence
☐ 4. Decreased ventricular wall compliance

CORRECT ANSWER: 4
S_3 results from increased resistance to ventricular filling, such as would occur in an MI. Option 1: This does not cause an S_3 sound. Option 2: S_3 is not a normal heart sound. Option 3: S_3 occurs because of a ventricular problem, not an atrial one.

NP: Assessment
CN: Physiological integrity
CNS: Physiological adaptation
CL: Analysis

---

114 A client is placed on home oxygen therapy, using a nasal cannula at 2 L/minute and an oxygen concentrator. The client expresses a fear of using oxygen at home, stating, "I just know it will blow up." What is the nurse's best response?

☐ 1. "That never happens anymore."
☐ 2. "Explain your feeling of fear to me further."
☐ 3. "Read this information I've given you, and you'll see you don't have anything to worry about."
☐ 4. "Thousands of people use oxygen therapy safely in the home."

CORRECT ANSWER: 2
Reflecting and clarification are therapeutic techniques. This response encourages exploration of the client's feelings. Options 1 and 4 dismiss the client's feelings. Option 3 would be useful only after the client's feelings are explored.

NP: Implementation
CN: Psychosocial integrity
CNS: Coping and adaptation
CL: Application

---

115 Which of the following instructions should the nurse plan to include when teaching diaphragmatic breathing to a client with COPD?

☐ 1. "Exhale slowly while leaning forward and pressing a pillow against your abdomen."
☐ 2. "Inhale and exhale slowly with your lips pursed."
☐ 3. "Use your incentive spirometer for 15 minutes twice daily."
☐ 4. "Breathe in slowly through your nose and exhale through your mouth. Repeat this deep breathing three times and then cough."

CORRECT ANSWER: 1
Manual pressure on the upper abdomen during exhalation trains and strengthens the diaphragm. Option 2 is an incorrect explanation of pursed-lip breathing. Option 3 promotes inspiratory muscle training only. Option 4 lists instructions for a preoperative and postoperative deep-breathing and coughing exercise.

NP: Planning
CN: Physiological integrity
CNS: Physiological adaptation
CL: Application

116 Which of the following would be the best preoperative nursing diagnosis for a client with a detached retina?

☐ 1. Anxiety related to loss of vision and potential failure to regain vision
☐ 2. Risk for infection related to the eye injury
☐ 3. Pain related to tissue injury and decreased circulation to the eye
☐ 4. Knowledge deficit (preoperative and postoperative activities) related to lack of information

CORRECT ANSWER: 1
A client who perceives a threat to vision, such as a sudden loss of sight, is likely to be anxious. Because severe anxiety impairs the client's ability to process new information, it must be addressed before preoperative teaching. Option 2: The risk of infection is greater after surgery. Option 3: Pain would not be present preoperatively. Option 4: The client's anxiety must be dealt with before teaching is possible.

NP: Assessment
CN: Physiological integrity
CNS: Reduction of risk potential
CL: Analysis

---

117 A client is being treated for glaucoma with timolol (Timoptic) eyedrops. Which of the following statements by the client indicates proper understanding of the treatment?

☐ 1. "I must take this medication for the rest of my life to prevent my eyesight from becoming worse."
☐ 2. "I must take this medication until my symptoms are relieved."
☐ 3. "I must take this medication when I have headaches and blurred vision."
☐ 4. "I must stop this medication when I have used all of the bottle."

CORRECT ANSWER: 1
Lifelong therapy is required. The client should be instructed not to discontinue the medication without the physician's approval. Options 2, 3, and 4: The medication should not be discontinued or taken only when symptoms are present.

NP: Evaluation
CN: Physiological integrity
CNS: Pharmacological and parenteral therapies
CL: Analysis

---

118 Which of the following should be included in a client's postoperative plan of care after a stapedectomy?

☐ 1. Assess for damage to the laryngeal nerve.
☐ 2. Maintain bed rest for 72 to 96 hours.
☐ 3. Assess for damage to the facial nerve.
☐ 4. Increase fluids to 2 to 3 L per shift.

CORRECT ANSWER: 3
The surgical procedure is performed in an area where the facial nerve (VII), the acoustic nerve (VIII), and the vagus nerve (X) may be damaged. The nurse observes for complications by assessing for facial nerve damage. Option 1: The laryngeal nerve is not at risk for damage. Option 2: The client is ambulating with assistance 1 to 2 days after surgery. Option 4: Although adequate hydration is always important, forcing fluids is unnecessary.

NP: Planning
CN: Physiological integrity
CNS: Reduction of risk potential
CL: Application

119 A client is scheduled for rhinoplasty to repair a nasal fracture in which displacement has caused an airway obstruction. Which of the following preoperative instructions must be given?

☐ 1. How to use a straw
☐ 2. How to effectively breathe through the mouth
☐ 3. How to change nasal packing
☐ 4. Not to look in a mirror

CORRECT ANSWER: 2

Nasal packing will be inserted to control bleeding, so the client needs instructions in mouth-breathing techniques. Option 1: The client will not be allowed to use a straw because the pressure created by sucking may initiate bleeding. Option 3: The client should not remove the nasal packing. Option 4: A client who wants to look in a mirror should be prepared to see an edematous face.

NP: Implementation
CN: Physiological integrity
CNS: Reduction of risk potential
CL: Application

---

120 A 72-year-old male client has had a laryngectomy and is learning esophageal speech. He is discouraged and depressed. Which nursing intervention would be most beneficial?

☐ 1. Give him literature on esophageal speech.
☐ 2. Arrange for a visit from a member of the Lost Chord Club.
☐ 3. Ask family members to call or visit more often.
☐ 4. Tell him that he is lucky the cancer has not metastasized and that he has a good prognosis.

CORRECT ANSWER: 2

New laryngectomy clients usually benefit from a visit with another individual with a laryngectomy. Support groups can strengthen coping mechanisms and help prevent feelings of isolation, which can lead to discouragement and depression. Option 1: This impersonal action does not give direct and immediate support. Option 3: Talking on the phone or communicating with several family members at once may be impossible for the client at this time and does not directly address the problem. Option 4: This dismisses the client's feelings.

NP: Implementation
CN: Psychosocial integrity
CNS: Coping and adaptation
CL: Analysis

121 A 28-year-old homeless man comes to the outpatient clinic complaining of night sweats, hemoptysis, and pleuritic chest pain. He is admitted to the pulmonary unit with a diagnosis of rule-out tuberculosis and the following orders: sputum × 3 for cytology; purified protein derivative (PPD), mumps, and coccidioidomycosis skin tests; chest X-ray; complete blood count; and respiratory secretion isolation. The PPD skin test, read at 48 hours, reveals 3/4″ (20 mm) of redness and 5/8″ (16 mm) of induration around the injection site. The nurse interprets this information to indicate which of the following?

- ☐ 1. The client has a normal PPD test reaction.
- ☐ 2. The client is a PPD converter.
- ☐ 3. The client has been exposed to *Mycobacterium tuberculosis.*
- ☐ 4. The client has active tuberculosis.

CORRECT ANSWER: 3
An abnormal reaction indicates that a client has been exposed to *Mycobacterium tuberculosis.* It does not necessarily mean that active disease is present. More than 90% of tuberculin-significant reactors will not develop clinical tuberculosis. Option 1: This is an abnormal PPD. Option 2: No evidence suggests that the client had a normal reaction on a previous test. Option 4: This cannot be determined by a PPD. Sputum culture and chest X-ray are used to make this diagnosis.

NP: Assessment
CN: Health promotion and maintenance
CNS: Prevention and early detection of disease
CL: Application

---

122 A client was admitted 3 days ago with a suspected brain tumor. During assessment, the nurse notes clear drainage from the nose. Which of the following actions should the nurse take to determine whether the drainage is CSF?

- ☐ 1. Test for pH of the drainage.
- ☐ 2. Test for specific gravity of the drainage.
- ☐ 3. Test for glucose in the drainage.
- ☐ 4. Observe the drainage for a brown stain.

CORRECT ANSWER: 3
CSF has a high glucose content and therefore would test positive for sugar. Options 1 and 2: These are not specific tests for CSF identification. Option 4: Brown staining is not typical of CSF.

NP: Evaluation
CN: Physiological integrity
CNS: Physiological adaptation
CL: Application

---

123 A client with type 1 diabetes has had many renal calculi over the past 20 years and has now developed chronic renal failure. Which of the following must be reduced in planning the client's diet?

- ☐ 1. Carbohydrates
- ☐ 2. Fats
- ☐ 3. Protein
- ☐ 4. Vitamin C

CORRECT ANSWER: 3
Because of damage to the nephrons, the kidney cannot excrete all of the metabolic wastes of protein. Therefore, protein intake must be restricted. Options 1 and 2: Higher intake of carbohydrates and fats, together with vitamin supplements, are needed to ensure growth and maintenance of tissues. Option 4: Restricting vitamin C in this client's diet is unwarranted.

NP: Planning
CN: Physiological integrity
CNS: Basic care and comfort
CL: Application

124 A 28-year-old female is admitted to the hospital with a diagnosis of hepatitis B. She expresses concern about the duration of her recovery. Which of the following responses by the nurse is inappropriate?

- ☐ 1. Encourage her to express her feelings about the illness.
- ☐ 2. Provide avenues for financial counseling if she expresses the need.
- ☐ 3. Encourage her not to worry about the future.
- ☐ 4. Discuss the effects of hepatitis B on future health problems.

CORRECT ANSWER: 3

Telling the client to stop worrying minimizes her feelings and is an unrealistic goal. Option 1: Expressing her feelings will help the client. Option 2: If finances are a concern, then this is an appropriate response. Option 4: This is useful information for the client.

NP: Evaluation
CN: Psychosocial integrity
CNS: Coping and adaptation
CL: Application

---

125 A 50-year-old man is admitted to the hospital with a diagnosis of left lower lobe pneumonia. The physician orders ABG analysis, blood and sputum cultures, and 1 g of nafcillin (Unipen) I.V. every 4 hours. After the nurse explains the procedure for obtaining a sputum specimen, the client states, "I don't have anything to cough up right now." What should the nurse do next?

- ☐ 1. Ask him to try again later.
- ☐ 2. Suction the client to obtain the specimen.
- ☐ 3. Administer the first dose of nafcillin, and notify the physician.
- ☐ 4. Induce sputum with an aerosol treatment per hospital protocol.

CORRECT ANSWER: 4

Sputum production usually can be induced with an aerosol treatment. Option 1: Asking the client to try later may unduly delay treatment. Option 2: Suctioning the client will be traumatic for him if he has an effective cough and there is no sputum in the larger airways to suction out. Option 3: Antibiotics should not be administered until after cultures are obtained.

NP: Implementation
CN: Physiological integrity
CNS: Reduction of risk potential
CL: Application

---

126 A 58-year-old man is brought to the ED complaining of chest pain and light-headedness. He has a history of stable angina pectoris. An ECG is performed and a blood sample taken. Which part of the ECG complex should the nurse examine to determine active myocardial ischemia?

- ☐ 1. P wave
- ☐ 2. QRS complex
- ☐ 3. ST segment
- ☐ 4. U wave

CORRECT ANSWER: 3

The ST segment will be displaced in response to active myocardial ischemia. Option 1: The P wave measures atrial activity. Option 2: The QRS complex measures ventricular activity. Option 4: The U wave is only occasionally present and does not indicate ischemia.

NP: Assessment
CN: Physiological integrity
CNS: Physiological adaptation
CL: Analysis

127 A client has had a subtotal thyroidectomy. Which set of physician's orders should the nurse anticipate when the client returns from surgery to the medical-surgical unit?

☐ 1. Vital signs every 4 hours, flat supine position, nothing by mouth, strict intake and output

☐ 2. Vital signs every hour until stable, Trendelenburg's position, liquid diet, mist inhalation

☐ 3. Vital signs every 15 minutes until stable, semi-Fowler's position, fluids as tolerated, tracheostomy set at bedside

☐ 4. Vital signs every 2 hours, lateral recumbent position, house diet

CORRECT ANSWER: 3

Because hemorrhage and respiratory obstruction may develop, the nurse must take vital signs every 15 minutes until the client is stable, and then every 30 minutes to 1 hour for the next several hours. Options 1, 2, and 4: Vital signs must be checked more frequently. Furthermore, a flat supine position (Option 1) makes breathing more difficult, Trendelenburg's position (Option 2) is absolutely contraindicated, and it is too soon for the client to eat a house diet (Option 4).

NP: Planning
CN: Physiological integrity
CNS: Reduction of risk potential
CL: Application

---

128 The physician prescribes pyridostigmine bromide (Mestinon) four times daily for a client with myasthenia gravis. Which of the following times would be most appropriate for administration?

☐ 1. Before meals and upon awakening

☐ 2. After meals and at bedtime

☐ 3. Every 6 hours

☐ 4. According to the hospital medication schedule

CORRECT ANSWER: 1

Anticholinesterase agents must be taken according to an exact schedule and before expected times of energy consumption, such as before meals and upon awakening, to prevent respiratory and chewing difficulties. Option 2: The medication should be taken before meals. Options 3 and 4: These schedules might not ensure administration before energy-consuming activities.

NP: Planning
CN: Physiological integrity
CNS: Pharmacological and parenteral therapies
CL: Application

---

129 A client has been diagnosed with open-angle glaucoma. The physician's orders include one drop of pilocarpine hydrochloride (Pilocar) 1% in each eye, every 6 hours. Which instruction should the nurse provide the client?

☐ 1. Measure eye pressure once a day to determine if the medication is working.

☐ 2. Place one drop of medication in the inner canthus of each eye.

☐ 3. Notify the physician if the drops blur vision.

☐ 4. Refrain from driving at night.

CORRECT ANSWER: 4

Miotics constrict the pupils, inducing temporary blurred vision and impaired night vision. Option 1: The client has no way of measuring eye pressure. Option 2: The medication should be placed in the lower lid, with a finger pressed against the inner canthus to prevent systemic absorption. Option 3: Blurred vision is an expected adverse effect of miotics.

NP: Implementation
CN: Physiological integrity
CNS: Pharmacological and parenteral therapies
CL: Application

130 The nurse is evaluating a client after an injection of edrophonium (Tensilon). Which finding would confirm the diagnosis of myasthenia gravis?

☐ 1. Weakened respiratory inspiration
☐ 2. Increased LOC
☐ 3. Immediate improvement in muscular strength
☐ 4. Increased ptosis of the eyelid

CORRECT ANSWER: 3
Edrophonium facilitates transmission of nerve-muscle impulses, which is impaired in myasthenia gravis. Improved neuromuscular transmission will immediately increase muscle strength in clients with this disorder. Respiration (Option 1) and ptosis (Option 4) would improve after the client receives the drug. Option 2: Edrophonium should not affect one's LOC.

NP: Evaluation
CN: Physiological integrity
CNS: Pharmacological and parenteral therapies
CL: Analysis

---

131 A client with otosclerosis is admitted to the hospital for a complete stapedectomy with prosthesis. Which of the following would be most important for the nurse to assess before surgery?

☐ 1. Symptoms of external otitis media
☐ 2. Conductive hearing loss
☐ 3. A family history of otosclerosis
☐ 4. Sensorineural hearing loss

CORRECT ANSWER: 1
To prevent introduction of infective material into the middle-ear structures, the client must be free from external ear infection at the time of surgery. Option 2: Although conductive hearing loss may be present, this has no direct bearing on the client's surgical outcome. Option 3: A family history of otosclerosis is not significant to the surgical outcome. Option 4: Sensorineural hearing loss is not relevant to this situation.

NP: Assessment
CN: Physiological integrity
CNS: Reduction of risk potential
CL: Application

---

132 Which of the following should the nurse emphasize in discharge teaching of a young athlete with type 1 diabetes?

☐ 1. Reduce daily workouts and social activities.
☐ 2. Adjust carbohydrate intake and insulin administration to correlate with exercise.
☐ 3. Increase intake of protein and fats as energy sources.
☐ 4. Take additional insulin on days of planned exercise.

CORRECT ANSWER: 2
Persons with type 1 diabetes should increase their intake of carbohydrates before prolonged exercise. Option 1: With adequate carbohydrate intake, the client need not reduce exercise or social activity. Option 3: A balanced diabetic diet includes protein and fats, but carbohydrates provide the primary source of energy. Option 4: Taking extra insulin increases the risk of hypoglycemia.

NP: Planning
CN: Physiological integrity
CNS: Pharmacological and parenteral therapies
CL: Application

133 A client has just had an open reduction and casting of a forearm fracture. Which symptom of impending compartment syndrome should the nurse assess for?

- ☐ 1. Pain
- ☐ 2. Pallor
- ☐ 3. Paresthesia
- ☐ 4. Paralysis

CORRECT ANSWER: 1

Pain is the earliest and most significant symptom of compartment syndrome. Options 2, 3, and 4: Pallor, paresthesia, and paralysis occur later.

NP: Assessment
CN: Physiological integrity
CNS: Reduction of risk potential
CL: Application

---

134 A male client with rheumatoid arthritis explains that he still feels extreme pain in his joints, despite following all instructions. He doesn't see any point in trying anymore. What is the nurse's best response?

- ☐ 1. Ask the client to precisely describe his home regimen.
- ☐ 2. Listen attentively to his frustration about the chronic nature of his disease.
- ☐ 3. Suggest that a psychiatrist can help him cope better with his chronic illness.
- ☐ 4. Reassure him that he will improve if he continues the regimen.

CORRECT ANSWER: 2

Clients with rheumatoid arthritis usually feel frustrated; simply listening can diffuse some of their frustration. Option 1: Rheumatoid arthritis is a chronic disease that may not improve, even if the client does follow the recommended regimen. Option 3: Early referral to a psychiatrist is not indicated for a client experiencing normal frustration. Option 4: This provides false reassurance; improvement may not occur no matter what the client does.

NP: Implementation
CN: Psychosocial integrity
CNS: Coping and adaptation
CL: Application

---

135 A client with a comminuted fracture of the left femur becomes restless, confused, and irritable on the 2nd day in the hospital. Which of the following conditions should the nurse be alert for when assessing the client's symptoms?

- ☐ 1. Infection
- ☐ 2. Hyperthyroidism
- ☐ 3. Fat emboli syndrome
- ☐ 4. Anaphylactic shock

CORRECT ANSWER: 3

Fat emboli syndrome, a common complication after comminuted fractures of long bones, presents with these symptoms. Option 1: Infection is unlikely to create these symptoms, particularly confusion. Option 2: Symptoms do not suggest hyperthyroidism at this time. Option 4: These are not typical symptoms of anaphylactic shock.

NP: Assessment
CN: Safe, effective care environment
CNS: Physiological adaptation
CL: Analysis

136 A client who underwent a lung lobectomy the day before has anterior chest tubes connected to an underwater seal with suction. The nurse notices no bubbling in the suction compartment. What should the nurse do next?

- ☐ 1. Try milking the chest tube in slow, even strokes.
- ☐ 2. Add more sterile water to the suction compartment.
- ☐ 3. Check the physician's order for the amount of suction and increase the suction pressure until gentle bubbling can be seen.
- ☐ 4. Check the physician's order for the amount of suction and increase the water seal by 4″ (10 cm).

CORRECT ANSWER: 3

A chest tube attached to suction should have continuous gentle bubbling in the suction compartment to ensure proper functioning. Option 1 will not address a problem with suction. Option 2 will not correct the problem and could create other problems. Option 4 is unsafe.

NP: Implementation
CN: Safe, effective care environment
CNS: Safety and infection control
CL: Analysis

---

137 The nurse is planning discharge for a client who has had a stapedectomy. Which of the following should the nurse consider when planning care?

- ☐ 1. The client will not be allowed to go up and down stairs.
- ☐ 2. The client will need to have a daily shower.
- ☐ 3. The client must refrain from taking car rides for 6 weeks.
- ☐ 4. The client is at risk for falling.

CORRECT ANSWER: 4

The persistent vertigo that occurs after stapedectomy puts the client in danger of falling. Option 1: The client may go up and down stairs with assistance. Option 2: The client should avoid showering and getting the head and wound wet. Option 3: The client may ride in a car.

NP: Planning
CN: Physiological integrity
CNS: Physiological adaptation
CL: Application

---

138 A female client with a history of pulmonary edema calls the clinic complaining of shortness of breath, coughing, bloody mucus, and chest pain. What is the best nursing intervention?

- ☐ 1. Tell the client to lie down and rest.
- ☐ 2. Tell the client you will visit as soon as you can for further assessment.
- ☐ 3. Instruct the client to increase her oxygen concentration from 2 to 4 L.
- ☐ 4. Instruct the client to hang up, call 911, and have an ambulance bring her to the hospital.

CORRECT ANSWER: 4

The client's signs and symptoms indicate a recurrence of pulmonary edema, a life-threatening situation that requires immediate intervention. Options 1 and 2: Intervention cannot wait; the situation may be life-threatening. Option 3: Increasing oxygen will not be effective with increased lung secretions. The situation is life-threatening and calls for immediate medical attention.

NP: Implementation
CN: Physiological integrity
CNS: Physiological adaptation
CL: Application

139 Which of the following statements by a client taking nitroglycerin (Nitrostat) would indicate the need for additional teaching before discharge?

☐ 1. "I will renew my nitroglycerin supply every 6 months and discard any tablets I have that are over 6 months old."

☐ 2. "I will carry my nitroglycerin with me at all times in a dark-colored glass bottle."

☐ 3. "I will discard my nitroglycerin if it causes a burning sensation under my tongue because this indicates that the drug is stale."

☐ 4. "After I place the nitroglycerin tablet under my tongue, I will try not to swallow until the tablet dissolves."

CORRECT ANSWER: 3

A burning sensation under the tongue indicates that the nitroglycerin tablets are fresh. Option 1: A client's supply of nitroglycerin should be renewed every 6 months and old tablets discarded. Option 2: Nitroglycerin is inactivated by heat, moisture, air, light, and time. Because of this, the client should carry a supply of nitroglycerin in an airtight, dark glass container. Clients with angina should carry a supply of nitroglycerin at all times. Option 4: Gastric secretions may inactivate nitroglycerin; therefore, the client should let the sublingual tablet dissolve completely before swallowing.

NP: Evaluation
CN: Physiological integrity
CNS: Pharmacological and parenteral therapies
CL: Analysis

---

140 A 65-year-old client is admitted for a femoropopliteal bypass graft of the left leg. Which postoperative goal would take priority?

☐ 1. Prevent graft occlusion.

☐ 2. Prevent infection at the graft site.

☐ 3. Relieve postoperative pain.

☐ 4. Maintain adequate fluid balance.

CORRECT ANSWER: 1

Prevention and detection of graft occlusion is the first and foremost concern. The nurse should assess pulses every 15 minutes for the first hour and thereafter every hour. The nurse should also assess skin color, temperature, and pain and immediately report loss of pulses to the physician. Options 2, 3, and 4 are important, but prevention of graft occlusion is the primary concern after this type of surgery.

NP: Planning
CN: Physiological integrity
CNS: Pharmacological and parenteral therapies
CL: Analysis

---

141 Which of the following statements made by a client with pneumonia indicates proper understanding about preventing a recurrence?

☐ 1. "I will wear a face mask when walking in cold weather."

☐ 2. "My used tissues will be put in a bag that will be burned."

☐ 3. "I will drink 2 L of fluid per day."

☐ 4. "I will get my influenza vaccine at the prescribed time."

CORRECT ANSWER: 4

Once a person is initially exposed to pneumonia, a recurrence is more likely. The influenza vaccine is administered to prevent the development of a respiratory infection. Option 1: Face masks are used to prevent exercise-induced asthma. Option 2: Used tissues are burned to prevent the spread of TB. Option 3: Drinking lots of fluids will thin respiratory secretions.

NP: Evaluation
CN: Health promotion and maintenance
CNS: Prevention and early detection of disease
CL: Analysis

142 An 18-year-old male has fractured his spine at the level of the sixth cervical vertebrae in a diving accident. Initially, what is the best position for the client?

☐ 1. Prone, with the head to the side
☐ 2. Side lying, with the head midline
☐ 3. High Fowler's, with the head to the side
☐ 4. Supine, with the head midline

CORRECT ANSWER: 4

The best initial position for a person with a cervical fracture is supine, with the head immobilized and midline. This prevents flexion, rotation, and extension of the neck. Options 1 and 3: Turning the head could further injure the spine and diminish neurologic function. Option 2: After immobilization of the head and neck, the client may be logrolled. However, the client should not remain on his side. After cervical tongs are in place, he will usually be placed on a Stryker or Foster frame and turned from prone to supine.

NP: Implementation
CN: Physiological integrity
CNS: Physiological adaptation
CL: Application

---

143 A client is in the ED with a diagnosis of inferior-wall MI caused by an embolism. The physician has prescribed streptokinase (Streptase) I.V. What is the most important drug-induced adverse effect for the nurse to assess for during administration?

☐ 1. Cardiac arrhythmias
☐ 2. Symptoms of bleeding
☐ 3. Increased chest pain
☐ 4. Symptoms of pulmonary edema

CORRECT ANSWER: 2

Streptokinase promotes systemic thrombolysis by activating plasminogen, which degrades all fibrin clots. Option 1: The client should be observed for arrhythmias because of MI, not because of streptokinase administration. Option 3: Increased chest pain may indicate an extension of the infarct; it would not result from the streptokinase. Option 4: Pulmonary edema is not a response to streptokinase.

NP: Implementation
CN: Physiological integrity
CNS: Pharmacological and parenteral therapies
CL: Application

---

144 A client who has suffered a closed head injury is difficult to arouse and is experiencing 10-second periods of apnea. The physician orders intubation and mechanical ventilation. After 1 hour of mechanical ventilation, the following ABG values are obtained: pH, 7.47; $Paco_2$, 28; HCO_3-, 23. What condition do these results indicate?

☐ 1. Respiratory acidosis
☐ 2. Respiratory alkalosis
☐ 3. Metabolic acidosis
☐ 4. Metabolic alkalosis

CORRECT ANSWER: 2

Elevated pH and decreased $Paco_2$ indicate respiratory alkalosis. This is desirable in clients with closed head injuries because it lowers ICP. Option 1: In respiratory acidosis, pH is less than 7.35 and $Paco_2$ is elevated. Option 3: In metabolic acidosis, pH is less than 7.35 and HCO_3- is less than 22. Option 4: In metabolic alkalosis, pH is greater than 7.45 and HCO_3- is elevated.

NP: Evaluation
CN: Physiological integrity
CNS: Physiological adaptation
CL: Analysis

145 A male client with active TB is admitted to the nursing unit. Which action should the nurse take to prevent the spread of the tubercle bacillus?

☐ 1. Wear a gown and mask when caring for the client.
☐ 2. Teach the client how to cover his nose and mouth when coughing or sneezing.
☐ 3. Recommend that the client wear a mask when in contact with others.
☐ 4. Initiate body secretion precautions.

CORRECT ANSWER: 2
TB is transmitted by inhalation of tubercle-laden droplets. Client teaching includes covering the nose and mouth with disposable tissues when coughing or sneezing. Options 1 and 4 are unnecessary. Option 3 should not be necessary unless the client cannot comply with the less restrictive precautions.
NP: Planning
CN: Physiological integrity
CNS: Reduction of risk potential
CL: Application

---

146 Two hours after a left-sided lung lobectomy, a client returns from surgery with a chest tube connected to a water-seal chest drainage system. Fluctuation in the water-seal chamber stops, and breath sounds remain diminished in the left lung fields. What is the most probable cause?

☐ 1. A pleural leak is present.
☐ 2. The suction is too high.
☐ 3. The lung has reexpanded.
☐ 4. An obstruction is present.

CORRECT ANSWER: 4
Chest tubes drain fluid and remove air and can become plugged by blood clots, fibrin, or kinking. This obstruction will halt the normal fluctuation in the water-seal chamber. Option 1: A pleural leak is indicated by rapid and constant bubbling in the water-seal chamber. Option 2: Bubbling in the suction-control chamber indicates the presence of suction. Option 3: The client's diminished breath sounds indicate lack of air in the left lung. The lung will not reexpand for 24 hours to several days, depending on the cause of the pneumothorax.
NP: Evaluation
CN: Physiological integrity
CNS: Physiological adaptation
CL: Analysis

---

147 A client with unstable angina and hypertension has a history of severe COPD. Which of the following prescribed medications should the nurse question before administering it to the client?

☐ 1. Isosorbide dinitrate (Isordil)
☐ 2. Nifedipine (Procardia)
☐ 3. Nitroglycerin (Nitrostat)
☐ 4. Propranolol hydrochloride (Inderal)

CORRECT ANSWER: 4
Propranolol hydrochloride is used cautiously in a client with COPD because it can increase airway resistance. Options 1 and 3: These antianginal agents are not contraindicated with COPD. Option 2: This calcium channel blocker is not contraindicated with COPD.
NP: Implementation
CN: Physiological integrity
CNS: Pharmacological and parenteral therapies
CL: Application

148 A client comes to the ED with thyroid storm. What should the nurse do first?

☐ 1. Administer a corticosteroid I.V. as ordered to inhibit the release of thyroid hormone.
☐ 2. Give the client a cool bath to reduce the body temperature.
☐ 3. Monitor intake and output.
☐ 4. Initiate an ordered I.V. for administration of fluids and medications.

Correct answer: 4

Thyroid storm is a medical emergency. All of the listed options will be carried out, but the I.V. line should be started first so that it will be available to administer prescribed fluids and medications. Option 1: A corticosteroid cannot be administered until the I.V. line is in place. Options 2 and 3: These are important, but the I.V. has first priority.

NP: Implementation
CN: Physiological integrity
CNS: Physiological adaptation
CL: Analysis

---

149 After a transsphenoidal hypophysectomy, a client must be monitored for CSF loss. Which of the following indicates active fluid loss?

☐ 1. The client is swallowing frequently.
☐ 2. The client has tachycardia.
☐ 3. The client has decreased visual acuity.
☐ 4. The clear drainage on the dressing forms a halo.

Correct answer: 4

CSF will leave a halo on the gauze as it collects. Options 1, 2, and 3 usually are not associated with CSF loss.

NP: Assessment
CL: Physiological integrity
CNS: Reduction of risk potential
CL: Application

---

150 The nurse is preparing to give a 60-year-old male diabetic his morning dose of regular insulin. Why does the nurse remove it from the refrigerator ½ hour before administration?

☐ 1. Regular insulin is cooled to reduce bacteria.
☐ 2. Administration of cold insulin promotes lipodystrophy.
☐ 3. Refrigeration of insulin destroys its therapeutic effect.
☐ 4. Cold insulin has a reduced duration of action.

Correct answer: 2

Lipodystrophy, a condition marked by lipoma-like accumulation beneath the skin, is a complication of insulin administration. Rotating injection sites and administering insulin at room temperature help prevent this. Options 1, 3, and 4 are inaccurate.

NP: Implementation
CN: Physiological integrity
CNS: Pharmacological and parenteral therapies
CL: Application

151 A client has returned to the surgical unit after having a rhinoplasty under local anesthesia. Which reason should the nurse give to the client for being placed in semi-Fowler's position?

☐ 1. To allow blood to flow down the throat
☐ 2. To prevent aspiration
☐ 3. To minimize edema
☐ 4. To prevent increased ICP

CORRECT ANSWER: 3
Semi-Fowler's position uses gravity to promote circulation from the operative site, thus minimizing edema. Option 1: Bleeding should be absent; therefore, blood should not be flowing down the throat. Option 2: Aspiration is not a concern because the client received local anesthesia and is awake. Option 4: ICP is not a concern after rhinoplasty.

NP: Implementation
CN: Physiological integrity
CNS: Reduction of risk potential
CL: Application

---

152 A 48-year-old male complains of severe substernal chest pain radiating down his left arm. Although the client has no history of chest pain, he is admitted to the coronary care unit with a diagnosis of MI and is placed on a cardiac monitor. His physician prescribes morphine sulfate to relieve the chest pain. Which of the following must the nurse confirm before administering the drug?

☐ 1. The client is truly experiencing chest pain.
☐ 2. The client is not experiencing constipation.
☐ 3. The client's respiratory rate is at least 12 breaths/minute.
☐ 4. The client is free from cardiac arrhythmias.

CORRECT ANSWER: 3
Respiratory depression is an adverse effect of morphine sulfate. Option 1: Pain is a subjective experience. Relief of chest pain in MI is a priority because anxiety related to unrelieved chest pain increases myocardial oxygen demand, which may result in further myocardial damage. Option 2: Constipation is a long-term adverse effect of morphine. Option 4: Cardiac arrhythmias are not an adverse effect of morphine.

NP: Assessment
CN: Physiological integrity
CNS: Pharmacological and parenteral therapies
CL: Application

---

153 An 80-year-old male is admitted to the hospital with pneumonia. The next day, he refuses to use his incentive spirometer, saying, "I am too old and too tired to care anymore. Just leave me alone!" What would be the nurse's best response?

☐ 1. "You are not too old."
☐ 2. "I don't like to hear talk like this."
☐ 3. "Let's not talk about being old; you have many years left."
☐ 4. "You seem very tired this morning. . . ."

CORRECT ANSWER: 4
This validates the client's feeling of frustration and invites further expression of his emotions. Option 1 negates the client's feelings. Option 2 belittles the client. Option 3 dismisses his feelings.

NP: Assessment
CN: Psychosocial integrity
CNS: Coping and adaptation
CL: Analysis

154 A client with COPD experiences worsening dyspnea. ABG results show the following values: pH, 7.26; $Paco_2$, 70 mm Hg; Pao_2, 65 mm Hg; and HCO_3-, 35 mEq/L. The physician has ordered oxygen therapy at 2 L/minute. What is the best rationale for the low-dose oxygen therapy?

- ☐ 1. COPD clients do not absorb oxygen as well as other clients because of damaged lung tissues.
- ☐ 2. For COPD clients, the stimulus to breathe is a low oxygen level.
- ☐ 3. To be effective, larger doses of oxygen would have to be delivered via a rebreathing mask.
- ☐ 4. Oxygen at higher concentrations would dry the nasal mucosa.

CORRECT ANSWER: 2

Because the COPD client has chronic elevated levels of carbon dioxide, low oxygen replaces high carbon dioxide as the stimulus for breathing. The borderline or diminished ventilatory drive of these clients may be further suppressed by increasing the level of oxygen therapy. Option 1: This would not be a reason to give low doses of oxygen. Option 3: A rebreathing mask would further increase the client's already-elevated $Paco_2$. Option 4: Although true, this is not the rationale for the use of low-dose oxygen therapy in COPD.

NP: Implementation
CN: Physiological integrity
CNS: Reduction of risk potential
CL: Application

---

155 Why are clients who take digoxin (Lanoxin) and furosemide (Lasix) at risk for developing a toxic reaction to a digitalis glycoside?

- ☐ 1. Furosemide tends to cause hyperkalemia.
- ☐ 2. Digoxin has negative chronotropic effects.
- ☐ 3. Digoxin has positive inotropic effects.
- ☐ 4. Furosemide tends to decrease the serum potassium level.

CORRECT ANSWER: 4

Loop diuretics commonly cause hypokalemia, which potentiates the toxic effects of digoxin. Option 1: Furosemide tends to cause hypokalemia, not hyperkalemia. Option 2: Digoxin slows the heart rate, but this does not increase the client's risk of a toxic reaction. Option 3: Digoxin increases the force of myocardial contractility, but this does not increase the client's risk of a toxic reaction.

NP: Implementation
CN: Physiological integrity
CNS: Pharmacological and parenteral therapies
CL: Application

---

156 A 78-year-old female has recently been discharged from the hospital after experiencing heart failure related to long-standing hypertension and coronary artery disease. As a home health nurse, you are visiting her to evaluate her compliance with medication therapy. The client states that she is tired of eating bananas. Which of the following foods could the nurse suggest as a substitute?

- ☐ 1. One cup of corn flakes
- ☐ 2. One cup of oatmeal
- ☐ 3. Two slices of whole wheat bread
- ☐ 4. A medium baked potato

CORRECT ANSWER: 4

A medium baked potato contains 407 mg of potassium; a banana has 451 mg of potassium. Option 1: One cup of corn flakes contains 26 mg of potassium. Option 2: One cup of oatmeal contains 99 mg of potassium. Option 3: Two slices of whole wheat bread contain 88 mg of potassium.

NP: Implementation
CN: Physiological integrity
CNS: Basic care and comfort
CL: Analysis

157 A 72-year-old female has been admitted to the same-day surgical unit for cataract extraction involving the left eye. She tells the nurse that she is afraid of feeling pain during surgery. What is the nurse's best response?

- ☐ 1. "You shouldn't worry; the doctor knows what he is doing."
- ☐ 2. "Lasers allow for painless surgical procedures."
- ☐ 3. "The nerves around the eye will be numbed so that you will not feel pain."
- ☐ 4. "You will be asleep throughout the surgical procedure."

CORRECT ANSWER: 3

A local anesthetic is used to paralyze the nerves around and behind the eye. Option 1: Telling the client not to worry does not provide the information and support needed to allay her concerns. Option 2: Lasers are not used to remove cataracts. Option 4: This operation is usually done under local anesthesia. The client may be sedated but should not be asleep.

NP: Implementation
CN: Physiological integrity
CNS: Reduction of risk potential
CL: Application

---

158 The nurse is caring for a client scheduled for a stapedectomy. The client remarks, "I can't wait until after the surgery when I can finally hear!" What is the best response by the nurse?

- ☐ 1. "Has the doctor explained the surgical procedure to you?"
- ☐ 2. "Noticeable improvement in hearing may take as long as 6 weeks after surgery."
- ☐ 3. "The success rate of this surgery is high, but you need to be ready to accept failure."
- ☐ 4. "You won't notice any improvement in hearing until after 24 hours, when the gelfoam ear packing is removed."

CORRECT ANSWER: 2

Clients should be told that noticeable improvement in hearing may take as long as 6 weeks after surgery. Hearing will be impaired until after the postoperative edema has been resolved. Option 1: This does not provide the specific information that the client should have. Option 3: This is an unnecessarily negative response. Option 4: Improvement cannot be expected this quickly.

NP: Implementation
CN: Physiological integrity
CNS: Reduction of risk potential
CL: Application

---

159 A client is receiving an I.V. theophylline (Aminophylline) drip to relieve bronchospasm secondary to pulmonary edema. Which of the following symptoms would suggest a toxic reaction to the drug?

- ☐ 1. Ventricular arrhythmias
- ☐ 2. Absent peripheral pulses
- ☐ 3. Confusion
- ☐ 4. Glucose in the urine

CORRECT ANSWER: 1

Ventricular arrhythmias are associated with theophylline levels greater than 35 mcg/ml. The therapeutic serum concentration of theophylline is 10 to 20 mcg/ml. Options 2, 3, and 4: These signs and symptoms are not associated with theophylline therapy.

NP: Evaluation
CN: Physiological integrity
CNS: Pharmacological and parenteral therapies
CL: Comprehension

160 A 64-year-old client with COPD is assigned to your unit. Oxygen is ordered via nasal cannula at 2 L/minute. When the nurse makes rounds, she finds that the client's respirations have increased since admission. He is dusky, and his skin is cool and clammy. Which of the following should the nurse do first?

☐ 1. Increase the oxygen to 10 L/minute.
☐ 2. Acknowledge the client's physical symptoms, and encourage him to express his feelings.
☐ 3. Check vital signs.
☐ 4. Prepare to place the client on a ventilator.

CORRECT ANSWER: 3

Increased respirations, cyanosis, and cool, clammy skin may indicate any one of several medical emergencies. Checking vital signs will give the nurse more information about the client's condition. Option 1: High levels of oxygen are contraindicated in clients with COPD, as the extra oxygen diminishes their hypoxic drive to breathe. Option 2: These measures are important once the client's condition has been stabilized; however, the client's physiologic need for increased gas exchange and perfusion should be addressed first. Option 4: Assessment should always be done on clients experiencing changes in condition before implementation.

NP: Implementation
CN: Physiological integrity
CNS: Physiological adaptation
CL: Application

Posttest

QUESTIONS

1 A 3-year-old client with sickle cell disease is admitted to the hospital in vaso-occlusive crisis. Which of the following nursing diagnostic categories should be given priority in her initial nursing plan of care?

- ☐ 1. Pain
- ☐ 2. Unilateral neglect
- ☐ 3. Fluid volume excess
- ☐ 4. Hypothermia

2 A 1-day-old infant is in the newborn nursery with a lumbosacral myelomeningocele. The myelomeningocele sac is intact and covered by a fluid-filled membrane. The client is lying prone and the sac is being kept moist and sterile with normal saline solution. Which of the following problems can the saline solution cause?

- ☐ 1. Increased fluid loss
- ☐ 2. Temperature instability
- ☐ 3. Infection
- ☐ 4. Diffusion of saline across the membrane

3 Which of the following should the nurse monitor in a client with Cushing's syndrome who is taking corticosteroids?

- ☐ 1. Weight, electrolyte levels, and intake and output
- ☐ 2. Diet for increased sodium and decreased potassium
- ☐ 3. Symptoms of hypoglycemia
- ☐ 4. Symptoms of fluid volume deficit

4 A 22-year-old female has been receiving chemotherapy for 2 months. She tells the nurse that she always experiences vomiting after receiving chemotherapy. Which administration time would be most helpful to the client when giving an antiemetic on an as-needed basis?

- ☐ 1. Just before chemotherapy
- ☐ 2. As soon as nausea is felt
- ☐ 3. As soon as vomiting begins
- ☐ 4. One hour after receiving chemotherapy

5 A $3^1/_2$-year-old child admitted to the pediatric unit with a diagnosis of abdominal pain is afebrile and not complaining of pain at this time. What is the best choice of activities when the nurse takes the child to the playroom?

- ☐ 1. A jigsaw puzzle with 200 pieces
- ☐ 2. A game of patty-cake
- ☐ 3. Quiet play alone with a bucket and shovel
- ☐ 4. Ring-around-a-rosy with a group of children

6 A 19-year-old primigravida is $2^1/_4$″ (6 cm) dilated. An epidural catheter is placed, and she receives a test dose and then an analgesic dose of epidural anesthetic. The nurse assesses her blood pressure frequently because hypotension is a common adverse effect of the anesthetic. Which of the following nursing actions can minimize the possibility of hypotension?

☐ 1. Administer oxygen.
☐ 2. Elevate the client's legs.
☐ 3. Prehydrate the client.
☐ 4. Use warmed blankets.

7 A 20-month-old client is scheduled for surgical correction of hypospadias in the outpatient surgical unit. Preoperative teaching is done by the office nurse. When should the client be told that he will receive a preoperative injection?

☐ 1. At the same time all other teaching is done
☐ 2. After his mother takes him home
☐ 3. When he first enters the hospital
☐ 4. Immediately before the injection is given

8 A baby boy was born at a gestational age of 39 weeks via normal, spontaneous delivery after 17 hours of oxytocin (Pitocin) induction. His Apgar score was 7 at 1 minute and 9 at 5 minutes. The baby is now 1 day old. Which of the following should the nurse monitor closely, considering the circumstances of his birth?

☐ 1. Hyperbilirubinemia
☐ 2. Hypoglycemia
☐ 3. Polycythemia
☐ 4. Hyperthermia

9 A nurse is assigned to care for a 39-year-old hyperactive, elated client who exhibits flight of ideas, eats poorly, and does not attend to personal hygiene. What should the nurse do to help the client with personal hygiene?

☐ 1. Restrict makeup because she will apply it too freely.
☐ 2. Suggest that she wear hospital clothing to avoid power struggles.
☐ 3. Give her the freedom to look and dress as she pleases.
☐ 4. Assist her with clothing choices and makeup application.

10 A nurse discovers that she has charted assessments on the wrong client's chart. Which corrective action should the nurse take?

☐ 1. Notify the supervisor immediately.
☐ 2. Carefully erase the incorrect entry.
☐ 3. Draw a line through the entry and write "error."
☐ 4. Black out the entire entry and record "written in error."

11 Which common adverse effect of chemotherapeutic drugs is most likely to cause problems with body image?

☐ 1. Alopecia
☐ 2. Bone marrow depression
☐ 3. Red-tinged urine
☐ 4. Nausea and vomiting

12 While planning a community screening to identify skin cancer, a nurse does research on melanoma. Which population group will the nurse focus on during assessment?

☐ 1. People eating a diet high in iodine
☐ 2. People eating high-fat, low-fiber diets
☐ 3. People with extensive exposure to sunlight
☐ 4. People living in urban areas

13 The nurse is helping a client with hyperthyroidism to select an appropriate diet. Which of the following would help provide adequate nutrition?

☐ 1. High protein and low calories
☐ 2. High protein and high calories
☐ 3. No between-meal snacks
☐ 4. Low fat and low carbohydrates

14 A 4-year-old boy is admitted to the hospital for chemotherapeutic treatment for acute lymphocytic leukemia. Which of the following sites should the nurse avoid when administering vesicant chemotherapeutic agents to the client?

☐ 1. Shallow veins
☐ 2. Central lines
☐ 3. Antecubital fossa
☐ 4. Veins in the midforearm

15 A 4-year-old girl is brought to the emergency department by her parents. They explain that she injured her arm when she caught it in the rails of the stairs. Physical examination reveals a fracture of the right distal humerus. The child has several bruises on her buttocks and back. The nurse suspects child abuse. The mother protests that she knows nothing of this abuse and suggests that "the staff is lying." Which of the following most likely explains the mother's behavior?

☐ 1. She is jealous of the attention her daughter is receiving.
☐ 2. She frequently fights with her daughter.
☐ 3. She is abused herself.
☐ 4. She is uninvolved with the child's care.

16 A 23-year-old architectural student is admitted to the intensive care unit with a blood pressure of 210/110 mm Hg. He is taking phenelzine (Nardil) and had eaten some lasagna at dinner. His family knows he takes medication for depression and is very concerned. The family asks the nurse what happened. What is the best response by the nurse?

☐ 1. "Don't worry; he will be all right."
☐ 2. "He is young and strong, and these two factors are on his side."
☐ 3. "Eating certain foods with his medication is dangerous. The cheese in the lasagna caused his blood pressure to rise."
☐ 4. "It sounds like you are concerned about your son. We are giving him blood pressure medication."

17 Which of the following assessment findings of a newborn should the nurse report to the physician?

☐ 1. Positive Babinski's reflex
☐ 2. Vernix in groin and neck creases
☐ 3. Positive Ortolani's sign
☐ 4. Positive Moro's reflex

18 A 15-year-old client who delivered a baby 3 days ago was discharged early and is being seen at home by the nurse on her 3rd postpartal day. She did not receive anesthesia or analgesia during labor and did not have an episiotomy. The client is bottle-feeding her newborn. Which of the following physical assessment findings should the nurse report to the physician?

☐ 1. A pulse rate of 60 beats/minute
☐ 2. Uterus firm three fingerbreadths below the umbilicus
☐ 3. Tiredness during the day
☐ 4. Frequent voiding of scant amounts and burning on urination

19 A client is admitted to the oncology unit for treatment for uterine cancer. Routine laboratory tests reveal a total white blood cell count below normal limits, with a marked reduction in the neutrophil count. The client's physician orders 300 mg of lithium carbonate (Lithonate) to be taken orally three times per day. When the drug is administered for the first time, the client's husband becomes angry and follows the nurse out into the hallway. He whispers loudly, "That drug is for crazy people. My wife has cancer!" Which of the following is the nurse's best response to the husband?

☐ 1. "We understand that your wife has cancer. This drug is being given for other purposes."
☐ 2. "Calm down. Would you like to talk about it?"
☐ 3. "You are angry because you think we don't know what's wrong with your wife?"
☐ 4. "I'm sorry you are upset. Let me explain why the doctor ordered lithium."

20 A client scheduled for a proctoscopy has an I.V. in place. An order for 5 mg of I.V. diazepam (Valium) is written to be administered on call from the GI laboratory. Which protocol should be followed when administering the diazepam?

☐ 1. Mix with 50 ml of dextrose 5% in water and administer over 15 minutes.
☐ 2. Administer I.V. rapidly to prevent the bloodstream from diluting the drug mixture.
☐ 3. Administer in the I.V. port closest to the vein.
☐ 4. Question the order because I.V. administration of diazepam is contraindicated.

21 A 10-year-old boy has sickle cell anemia. What is the best action for the nurse to take when planning his physical activity program?

- ☐ 1. Prevent the client from playing outdoors with his friends at school.
- ☐ 2. Discuss the client's need for increased fluids with his teachers.
- ☐ 3. Encourage the client to try out for the ice hockey team.
- ☐ 4. Give the client aspirin when he is in pain or has a fever.

22 A 7-year-old client with hemophilia is admitted for a workup. Which nursing diagnostic category applies to this client?

- ☐ 1. Altered nutrition: less than body requirements
- ☐ 2. Risk for injury
- ☐ 3. Ineffective thermoregulation
- ☐ 4. Unilateral neglect

23 A 6-year-old girl has been admitted to the hospital with a diagnosis of rheumatic fever. She is to remain on complete bed rest with activity restrictions. Why would the nurse restrict activity during the acute phase of the illness?

- ☐ 1. To prevent skin breakdown
- ☐ 2. To reduce the workload of the heart
- ☐ 3. To prevent pressure on tender joints
- ☐ 4. To promote the benefits of drug therapy

24 An obese 56-year-old type 2 diabetic patient questions the nurse about the use of "dietetic" foods. What is the nurse's best response?

- ☐ 1. "These foods can be used freely because they do not contain sugar."
- ☐ 2. "The diabetic diet does not require the use of special or dietetic foods."
- ☐ 3. "These foods are a good idea because they are less expensive and will stretch your shopping dollars."
- ☐ 4. "You can use whatever you like as long as it does not contain sugar."

25 A 36-year-old female has been admitted with a diagnosis of Addison's disease. The physician orders electrolyte, blood urea nitrogen (BUN), blood glucose, and corticotropin stimulation tests. Which of the following would the nurse expect to find when analyzing laboratory findings?

- ☐ 1. Hypoglycemia
- ☐ 2. Decreased BUN level
- ☐ 3. Elevated sodium level
- ☐ 4. Decreased potassium level

26 A 74-year-old man with a history of heart failure is admitted with acute pulmonary edema. He is intubated and placed on a mechanical ventilator. What is the best position for this client?

- ☐ 1. Trendelenburg's
- ☐ 2. High Fowler's
- ☐ 3. Supine
- ☐ 4. Right side lying

27 A client is scheduled to have a radioactive implant inserted for treatment for uterine cancer. She questions the nurse about restrictions that may be placed on her activities after the implant is inserted. What is the nurse's best response?

- ☐ 1. "There will be no restrictions on your activities after the implant is inserted."
- ☐ 2. "You will be restricted to this unit after the implant is inserted; however, you may have unlimited visitors."
- ☐ 3. "You will be placed on bed rest or restricted to your room, and visiting restrictions will be necessary while the implant is in place."
- ☐ 4. "You will have no limitations on your activities, but visits from pregnant women are discouraged while the implant is in place."

28 A physician prescribes an I.V. loading dose of theophylline followed by a continuous infusion of theophylline. Which of the following signs and symptoms of a toxic reaction should the nurse observe for when administering methylxanthine medications?

- ☐ 1. Hypoglycemia and urticaria
- ☐ 2. Tachypnea and tachycardia
- ☐ 3. Tachycardia and nausea
- ☐ 4. Diarrhea and hypokalemia

29 Which of the following points should a team leader consider when delegating work to team members in order to conserve time?

☐ 1. Assign unfinished work to other team members.

☐ 2. Explain to each team member what needs to be done.

☐ 3. Relinquish responsibility for the outcome of the work.

☐ 4. Assign each team member the responsibility to obtain dietary trays.

30 A mother brings a 6-year-old child to the nurse, complaining that the child is suddenly not hearing anything the mother says. On examination, the nurse notes tender, enlarged, warm cervical lymph nodes. What is the most likely explanation for this?

☐ 1. Local scalp infection common in children

☐ 2. Infection or inflammation distal to the site

☐ 3. Infection or inflammation secondary to otitis media

☐ 4. Some form of cancer

31 A 9-month-old girl received immunizations at 2 months and 4 months. Immunizations at the 6-month visit were deferred because the child was febrile. Which immunizations should be given at the 9-month visit?

☐ 1. Diphtheria-pertusis-tetanus (DPT) vaccine only

☐ 2. DPT, live oral poliovirus, and Haemophilus influenza type B (Hib) vaccines, because her schedule was interrupted and must be started over

☐ 3. None, because no immunizations are given at the 9-month visit

☐ 4. DPT and Hib vaccines

32 A client had a left mediolateral episiotomy during a normal delivery. The nurse is teaching her perineal care. Which of the following is the most important strategy to review with the client to prevent infection?

☐ 1. Use moist heat therapy, such as sitz baths, twice daily to aid healing.

☐ 2. Clean the perineum and change the pad at least once daily.

☐ 3. Wash hands before and after changing the perineal pad, and clean the perineum from front to back.

☐ 4. Apply anesthetic spray as needed.

33 A 29-year-old primigravida client is in labor at 39 weeks' gestation. At the beginning of the second stage of labor, she is starting to push. The nurse notices the leaking amniotic fluid change from clear to green-yellow. The client's contractions have slowed to once every 3 to 4 minutes, and she complains of a new burning, stinging pain in her perineum, which is beginning to bulge. Which sign or symptom requires immediate action?

☐ 1. Stinging, burning perineal pain

☐ 2. Decreased frequency of uterine contractions

☐ 3. Bulging perineum

☐ 4. Change in color of the amniotic fluid

34 A 42-year-old man convicted of extorting funds from his employer is committed to the hospital for psychiatric evaluation and treatment. The client impresses the admitting nurse with his knowledge of the stock market, attempts to "con" the nurse into investing money with him in a particular stock, and then becomes loud and argumentative when she refuses. What should the nurse do next?

☐ 1. Quietly and calmly inform the client that his request is inappropriate in the hospital setting.

☐ 2. Raise her voice to match the client's tone and volume.

☐ 3. Reconsider her refusal and agree to discuss the proposition later.

☐ 4. Ask him why he thinks she is an "easy mark."

35 A 55-year-old man is diagnosed with acute schizophrenia after being found running down an interstate highway in his pajamas. He is violently agitated and states that he is being pursued by demons. He is admitted to the psychiatric unit for observation. To control his highly agitated state, the physician prescribes 50 mg of chlorpromazine hydrochloride (Thorazine) three times daily.

Which of the following would indicate a therapeutic response to the drug?
- ☐ 1. The client walks incessantly up and down the hallway outside his room, mumbling to himself.
- ☐ 2. The client's blood pressure falls from 160/80 mm Hg on admission to 100/60 mm Hg after 3 days of therapy.
- ☐ 3. The client drinks two glasses of water, having previously refused to take any fluids.
- ☐ 4. The client sleeps 6 hours during the night.

36 The parents of a 9-year-old diabetic boy tell the nurse that he is very involved in sports. They ask if there is anything they should be concerned about because of his diabetes. What advice should the nurse give?
- ☐ 1. The client may need to increase insulin intake.
- ☐ 2. The client may need to decrease food intake.
- ☐ 3. The client may be at risk for hyperglycemia.
- ☐ 4. The client may be at risk for hypoglycemia.

37 A client had a modified radical mastectomy 1 month ago. Which of the following behaviors would indicate that she is having difficulty coping with her feelings after the mastectomy?
- ☐ 1. The client expresses grief over the lost body part.
- ☐ 2. The client can view her incision without disgust.
- ☐ 3. The client requests information about support groups.
- ☐ 4. The client acts disinterested in her appearance.

38 A 28-year-old woman is brought to the nursing unit after an adrenalectomy. Which of the following postoperative assessment data should the nurse focus on monitoring?
- ☐ 1. Level of consciousness and orientation
- ☐ 2. Serum cortisol and aldosterone levels
- ☐ 3. Blood pressure and nausea and vomiting
- ☐ 4. Glucose and vasopressin levels

39 Which food would be contraindicated for a client on a low-sodium diet?
- ☐ 1. Fresh peaches
- ☐ 2. Peanut butter
- ☐ 3. Roast beef
- ☐ 4. Boiled eggs

40 A client has experienced significant blood loss during a colon resection. A major postoperative concern is the development of shock. A urinary catheter is inserted to measure hourly urine output. Which urine output would suggest inadequate fluid replacement?
- ☐ 1. 100 ml/hour
- ☐ 2. 30 ml/hour
- ☐ 3. 50 ml/hour
- ☐ 4. 75 ml/hour

41 A 1-year-old with a cardiac defect resulting in heart failure is taking digoxin (Lanoxin) daily. When instructing the parents, the nurse reveals how they can tell when the child is getting too much digoxin. Which of the following would best alert the parents to a possible toxic reaction to digoxin?
- ☐ 1. The child refuses to eat.
- ☐ 2. The child sees yellow rainbows.
- ☐ 3. The child has fewer wet diapers.
- ☐ 4. The child has a pulse rate of 100 to 120 beats/minute.

42 A mother brings her 6-year-old daughter to the clinic with a sore throat and a fever of 103°F (39.4°C). The physician orders a throat culture and a 10-day course of amoxicillin (Amoxil) for strep throat. What is the most important nursing action before the client and her mother leave the clinic?
- ☐ 1. Help the mother make a chart to ensure that the child receives all of her amoxicillin as scheduled.
- ☐ 2. Have the mother demonstrate her technique for taking the child's temperature so that she will know when the amoxicillin has worked.
- ☐ 3. Explain to the mother not to force the child to take fluids while her throat is sore.
- ☐ 4. Suggest that the mother invite friends in to play with the child.

43 A client delivered a baby girl 24 hours ago. While performing a postpartal check, the nurse finds the client's uterus firm at the umbilicus and deviated to the right. What should be the nurse's next action?

☐ 1. Notify the physician immediately.
☐ 2. Place her hand on the client's abdomen, and push the uterus toward the midline.
☐ 3. Place the client in a left side-lying position.
☐ 4. Have the client attempt to void.

44 A female client is admitted to the psychiatric unit after slashing her wrists in response to breaking up with her boyfriend. She is diagnosed with borderline personality disorder. On her 1st day on the unit, she announces that a fellow patient is her new boyfriend. On the 2nd day, she loudly and angrily demands that the staff move her room closer to the man. What is the best nursing intervention for the client's behavior?

☐ 1. Oblige her request for a room change.
☐ 2. Ask the man how he feels about rooming closer to her.
☐ 3. Move both clients to opposite corridors.
☐ 4. Point out that hospital rules do not allow room changes for friendship reasons.

45 A client has been diagnosed with panic disorder. Relaxation techniques and behavioral modifications have not decreased the incidence of panic attacks. The nurse has been asked to participate in an interdisciplinary team conference to consider drug therapy. Which of the following drugs should the nurse be prepared to discuss to relieve the client's panic attacks?

☐ 1. Meprobamate (Equanil)
☐ 2. Diazepam (Valium)
☐ 3. Lorazepam (Ativan)
☐ 4. Alprazolam (Xanax)

46 A 30-year-old man is being discharged 5 days after a surgical reduction of a compound fracture of the fibula. Which statement by the client would indicate to the nurse the need for more teaching about discharge instructions?

☐ 1. "I should report any extreme pain in my leg to my doctor."
☐ 2. "I should keep the cast completely dry while bathing."
☐ 3. "I should keep my casted leg elevated when sitting to prevent swelling and pain."
☐ 4. "I can remove the cast after 5 days at home."

47 The nurse is assessing the client's knowledge about osteoarthritis. Which statement by the client indicates a need for further teaching?

☐ 1. "I understand that the doctor can try to relieve my symptoms but cannot cure me."
☐ 2. "I am going to ask the doctor to give me those gold treatments like my friend had for her arthritis."
☐ 3. "I asked my doctor to draw blood to see if I'm getting better, but the doctor explained to me that there really aren't any blood tests that will tell me that."
☐ 4. "I am going to try to lose weight and be careful with my joints to help decrease the pain."

48 A 2-year-old boy is admitted with a suspected diagnosis of Hirschsprung's disease (aganglionic megacolon). He is placed on a low-residue diet. Which of the following breakfasts would adhere to this diet?

☐ 1. Raisin bran and orange juice
☐ 2. Fried eggs and bacon
☐ 3. Cheerios and apple juice
☐ 4. Pancakes with sausages and milk

49 A 6-hour-old infant is being observed in the nursery. Which of the following would lead the nurse to suspect tracheoesophageal fistula?

☐ 1. Coughing, choking, and coarse crackles
☐ 2. Cyanosis, copious oral secretions, and choanal atresia
☐ 3. Cyanotic episodes, coughing, and choking
☐ 4. Cyanosis, coughing, and constipation

50 A 3-year-old had a hypospadias repair yesterday. He has a suprapubic catheter and an I.V. running. Which of the following rationales is appropriate for administering propantheline bromide (Pro-Banthine) on an as-needed basis?

☐ 1. To decrease the chance of infection at the suture line
☐ 2. To decrease the number of organisms in the urine
☐ 3. To prevent bladder spasms while the catheter is present
☐ 4. To increase urine flow from the kidney to the ureters

51 A 31-year-old primigravida at 41 weeks' gestation is admitted for oxytocin (Pitocin) induction of labor. An infusion of 10 U of oxytocin in 1,000 ml of lactated Ringer's solution is begun, piggyback, into a primary I.V. The initial infusion rate is set at 6 ml/hour. After $1\frac{1}{2}$ hours, the rate is increased to 24 ml/hour. What is the amount of oxytocin in milliunits (mU) delivered per minute at a rate of 24 ml/hour?

☐ 1. 1 mU/minute
☐ 2. 2 mU/minute
☐ 3. 3 mU/minute
☐ 4. 4 mU/minute

52 A client has an arteriovenous fistula for hemodialysis treatments. What is the best way for the nurse to check for patency of the fistula?

☐ 1. Pinch the fistula and note the speed of filling on release.
☐ 2. Palpate the fistula throughout its length to assess for a thrill.
☐ 3. Use a needle and syringe to aspirate blood from the fistula.
☐ 4. Check for capillary refill of the nail beds on that extremity.

53 A 40-year-old female is admitted to the hospital for management of Cushing's syndrome. The next morning, she complains to the nurse that she is upset about her recent weight gain, thinning of scalp hair, and the purple marks on her abdomen that she noticed this morning. What is the most appropriate nursing response?

☐ 1. Report these clinical signs to the physician immediately.
☐ 2. Explain to the client that these are all common signs of Cushing's syndrome.
☐ 3. Tell the client that these signs are insignificant and will disappear shortly.
☐ 4. Administer her sedative as needed to help her relax.

54 A client has suffered cardiac arrest. Cardiopulmonary resuscitation (CPR) is begun within 2 minutes. Which drug, if ordered, will be administered based on the arterial blood gas (ABG) results?

☐ 1. Calcium chloride
☐ 2. Epinephrine (Adrenalin)
☐ 3. Furosemide (Lasix)
☐ 4. Sodium bicarbonate

55 A client tells the psychiatric admitting nurse that he is "just taking a rest because the Queen of England ordered me to." Which should the nurse note on the intake interview form?

☐ 1. Altered thought content
☐ 2. Altered thought processes
☐ 3. Altered motor behavior
☐ 4. Altered mood

56 A client has been receiving radiation therapy for cancer. Which of the following adverse effects of external beam radiation therapy would the nurse anticipate in developing a plan of care?

☐ 1. Constipation
☐ 2. Hypothermia
☐ 3. Fatigue
☐ 4. Increased appetite

57 You are teaching a client who has type 2 diabetes mellitus. Which teaching should be emphasized?

☐ 1. Get 8 hours of sleep per night.
☐ 2. Eat 50% of the diet in the form of protein.
☐ 3. Exercise for 30 minutes three or four times weekly.
☐ 4. Visit the health care provider at least every year.

58 A 6-month-old girl with no previous health problems is brought to the ambulatory care clinic by her mother for a routine well-child appointment. During physiologic assessment of the child, the nurse discovers that the baby's pulse rate is 200 beats/minute. The child is awake and calm. What should the nurse do first in evaluating this measurement?

- ☐ 1. Ask the mother for further family history of cardiovascular disease.
- ☐ 2. Assess the child for developmental delay.
- ☐ 3. Compare this value with norms for the child's age-group and with readings taken on previous visits to the clinic.
- ☐ 4. Begin arrangements to send the child for echocardiography in order to assess her for cardiac defects.

59 A 49-year-old female is receiving internal radiation therapy for cervical cancer. Before the insertion of the radiation device, the nurse assesses the client's understanding of the treatment. Which statement by the client would indicate the need for more teaching?

- ☐ 1. "I know the nurses are always there, but they will probably just spend short times with me or call me on the intercom."
- ☐ 2. "I'll have a catheter in my bladder, so I won't have to go to the bathroom to urinate."
- ☐ 3. "Hygiene is very important, so I'll need a complete bath every day during the treatment."
- ☐ 4. "I'll have my family and friends call me rather than visit for the next couple of days."

60 A 3-year-old girl has been admitted to the pediatric unit with abdominal pain. She is afebrile and free from pain right now. The night of her admission, she wets the bed. Which of the following would best explain her bed-wetting?

- ☐ 1. She has a urinary tract infection.
- ☐ 2. She is frightened about being in the hospital.
- ☐ 3. This is normal for a child of her age.
- ☐ 4. She is developmentally delayed.

ANSWERS AND RATIONALES

1 CORRECT ANSWER: 1

Vaso-occlusive crisis is sometimes called "pain crisis" because of its painful symptoms. Pain management is a top priority. Option 2: No data indicate neglect. Option 3: Children in vaso-occlusive crisis need extra fluids. Option 4: Children in vaso-occlusive crisis are usually febrile, not hypothermic.

NP: Assessment
CN: Physiological integrity
CNS: Physiological adaptation
CL: Analysis
CA: Child nursing

2 CORRECT ANSWER: 2

Even normal infants have temperature instability. The wet normal saline solution cools quickly and covers a large body surface area; this increases temperature instability and the risk of hypothermia, which has serious consequences for infants. Options 1 and 3: Infants with myelomeningocele may suffer fluid losses and be prone to infection if the sac tears; the saline soaks help prevent this. Option 4: The saline solution does not diffuse across the sac membrane.

NP: Implementation
CN: Physiological integrity
CNS: Reduction of risk potential
CL: Application
CA: Child nursing

3 CORRECT ANSWER: 1

An excess of corticosteroids results in fluid volume excess, which must be monitored. Options 2, 3, and 4 are incorrect because they are just the opposite of what is expected in Cushing's syndrome.

NP: Assessment
CN: Physiological integrity
CNS: Reduction of risk potential
CL: Application
CA: Adult nursing

4 CORRECT ANSWER: 1
Antiemetic therapy is most useful if initiated before the emetic episode in order to suppress pathways that trigger vomiting. Options 2, 3, and 4 are too late to counteract the emetic episodes.
NP: Planning
CN: Physiological integrity
CNS: Pharmacological and parenteral therapies
CL: Application
CA: Adult nursing

5 CORRECT ANSWER: 4
Preschoolers enjoy repetitive, interactive, clearly structured games. Option 1: This is too complex. If preschoolers fail at activities, they tend to feel guilty. Efforts must be praised and failure avoided. Option 2: This would probably not hold a preschooler's interest; it would be more appropriate for a younger child. Option 3: Preschoolers enjoy interactive play more than solitary play.
NP: Implementation
CN: Health promotion and maintenance
CNS: Growth and development through the life span
CL: Analysis
CA: Child nursing

6 CORRECT ANSWER: 3
Hydration with 500 to 1,000 ml of I.V. fluid will increase blood volume and minimize the effects of generalized vasodilation that occurs with epidural administration. Options 1 and 2 are used after hypotension occurs, not as preventive measures. Option 4 could promote vasodilation and increase the possibility of hypotension.
NP: Implementation
CN: Physiological integrity
CNS: Reduction of risk potential
CL: Application
CA: Maternal-infant nursing

7 CORRECT ANSWER: 4
Injections are usually traumatic preoperative events for children. A toddler should be prepared for painful procedures just before they are done in order to avoid anxiety. Options 1, 2, and 3 allow too much time for the toddler to become anxious.
NP: Implementation
CN: Psychosocial integrity
CNS: Coping and adaptation
CL: Application
CA: Child nursing

8 CORRECT ANSWER: 1
Hyperbilirubinemia in the newborn is one of the complications of a prolonged oxytocin induction. Option 2: The risk of hypoglycemia occurs in the first few hours after birth. Option 3: Polycythemia is not a risk from the labor events. Option 4: Hypothermia is a more common risk after birth.
NP: Assessment
CN: Health promotion and maintenance
CNS: Growth and development through the life span
CL: Analysis
CA: Maternal-infant nursing

9 CORRECT ANSWER: 4
This preserves the client's dignity and self-esteem and promotes self-care within reasonable limits. Option 1: The client will need help with her makeup because she will probably tend to go to extremes with it. Option 2: This does not help her learn new and better ways to deal with situations. Option 3: This may set her up as a target of ridicule by other clients.
NP: Implementation
CN: Psychosocial integrity
CNS: Psychosocial adaptation
CL: Application
CA: Mental health nursing

10 CORRECT ANSWER: 3
A single line must be drawn through the entire entry and the notation "error" must be made. Option 1: The mistake does not need to be reported to the supervisor; the nurse may take independent action. Option 2: The chart is a legal document; nothing should ever be erased from it. Option 4: The incorrect entry should be legible. Blacking out the entry would not be acceptable.

NP: Implementation
CN: Safe, effective care environment
CNS: Management of care
CL: Application
CA: Adult nursing

11 Correct answer: 1
Alopecia (hair loss) can negatively affect self-image and self-concept. Option 2: This adverse effect can cause infection, bleeding, and anemia, but it is not as likely to have a direct effect on body image. Option 3: This indicates nephrotoxicity or hemorrhagic cystitis. Option 4: This causes great distress, but alopecia is more likely to have a direct effect on body image.
NP: Implementation
CN: Psychosocial integrity
CNS: Coping and adaptation
CL: Application
CA: Adult nursing

12 Correct answer: 3
Melanoma occurs at a high rate among those who spend a great deal of time outdoors, such as farmers and sailors. Other risk factors are fair complexion, blue eyes, light-colored hair, and freckles. Options 1, 2, and 4: No evidence has been found linking melanoma with diet or urban living.
NP: Assessment
CN: Health promotion and maintenance
CNS: Prevention and early detection of disease
CL: Application
CA: Adult nursing

13 Correct answer: 2
Clients with hyperthyroidism have increased metabolic requirements that are met by a diet high in protein, calories, and carbohydrates. Option 1: Hyperthyroid clients need a diet high in calories. Option 3: Hyperthyroid clients are encouraged to eat six meals daily to obtain sufficient calories. Option 4: Hyperthyroid clients need a diet high in carbohydrates to provide sufficient calories. Fat is not necessarily restricted in the diet.
NP: Planning
CN: Physiological integrity
CNS: Basic care and comfort
CL: Application
CA: Adult nursing

14 Correct answer: 3
Because of the risk of tissue damage, vesicant agents should not be injected near a joint, such as the wrist or antecubital fossa. Option 1: Shallow veins are acceptable because infiltration is easily detected. Option 2: A central line reduces the incidence of tissue damage because infiltration is unlikely and the medication is diluted in a large volume of blood. Option 4: This is not contraindicated.
NP: Implementation
CN: Physiological integrity
CNS: Pharmacological and parenteral therapies
CL: Application
CA: Child nursing

15 Correct answer: 4
Individuals who raise a child with an abusive partner commonly distance themselves to help support denial. Option 1: This is more commonly related to sexual abuse. Options 2 and 3: Not enough data exist to support these conjectures.
NP: Assessment
CN: Psychosocial integrity
CNS: Psychosocial adaptation
CL: Application
CA: Mental health nursing

16 Correct answer: 3
Foods rich in tyramine, such as the aged cheese used in lasagna, should not be eaten by clients taking a monoamine oxidase inhibitor, such as phenelzine. The combination causes excessive norepinephrine release at the receptor site, precipitating a hypertensive crisis. Options 1 and 2: These responses give the family false reassurance and do not respond to the family's request for information. Option 4: This response expresses concern for the family and suggests a specific treatment, but it does not answer the family's request for information.
NP: Implementation
CN: Psychosocial integrity
CNS: Coping and adaptation
CL: Application
CA: Mental health nursing

17 Correct answer: 3

A positive Ortolani's sign indicates a congenital hip dislocation. Options 1, 2, and 4 are normal in the newborn.

NP: Assessment
CN: Health promotion and maintenance
CNS: Growth and development through the life span
CL: Application
CA: Maternal-infant nursing

18 Correct answer: 4

These complaints indicate a urinary tract infection, which would require a confirming diagnosis and appropriate antibiotic therapy. Option 1: Bradycardia is typical in the postpartal client, a result of the increased cardiac output and stroke volume demanded during pregnancy. Option 2: This would be expected, as the uterus generally involutes at a rate of one fingerbreadth per day. Option 3: This is a typical complaint of postpartal clients, especially with the newborn waking up at night. The mother should be encouraged to rest when the baby does.

NP: Assessment
CN: Physiological integrity
CNS: Physiological adaptation
CL: Analysis
CA: Maternal-infant nursing

19 Correct answer: 4

This acknowledges and accepts the husband's anger and offers concrete information to clarify the misunderstanding. Lithium carbonate is given to clients with cancer who have low neutrophil counts. However, the lay public is most familiar with the use of lithium in the treatment of bipolar depression. The husband's angry response is probably rooted in the anxiety he feels about his wife's medical diagnosis. The caregiver's first objective is to help clarify the immediate misunderstanding in order to establish trust so that the husband's underlying feelings of helplessness and anxiety about his wife's condition can be managed. Option 1: This response is defensive in tone and does not give the husband the full explanation he needs. Option 2: This response is belittling and potentially counterproductive because it invites the husband to refuse to discuss the issue. Option 3: This is a defensive restatement of the person's communication.

NP: Implementation
CN: Physiological integrity
CNS: Pharmacological and parenteral therapies
CL: Analysis
CA: Mental health nursing

20 Correct answer: 3

Diazepam is absorbed by the plastic I.V. tubing and should be given in the port closest to the vein. Option 1: Diazepam should not be mixed with any other solution or drug. Option 2: Diazepam should be administered slowly to avoid excessive central nervous system depression. Option 4: I.M. administration of diazepam is contraindicated because it is very painful as an injection.

NP: Implementation
CN: Physiological integrity
CNS: Pharmacological and parenteral therapies
CL: Comprehension
CA: Adult nursing

21 Correct answer: 2

Maintaining hydration is necessary to prevent a vaso-occlusive crisis. Option 1: This negates normalization of the boy's life and limits interaction with his peer group. Option 3: This sport is not recommended because vigorous exercise and cold stress can precipitate a vaso-occlusive crisis. Option 4: Use of aspirin is not recommended for a child with fever because of the risk of Reye's syndrome, and it is controversial for children in pain who have sickle cell anemia.

NP: Planning
CN: Physiological integrity
CNS: Reduction of risk potential
CL: Application
CA: Child nursing

22 Correct answer: 2

The increased potential for injury in those with hemophilia relates to a deficiency of the clotting factor. Options 1, 3, and 4 are not anticipated problems in clients with hemophilia.

NP: Analysis
CN: Physiological integrity
CNS: Reduction of risk potential
CL: Analysis
CA: Child nursing

23 CORRECT ANSWER: 2
As activity increases, the workload of the heart increases. Straining the heart increases the likelihood of carditis. Options 1, 3, and 4: Activity restriction will not in itself prevent skin breakdown, relieve joint pressure, or enhance the effects of drug therapy.
NP: Implementation
CN: Physiological integrity
CNS: Reduction of risk potential
CL: Application
CA: Child nursing

24 CORRECT ANSWER: 2
The standard diabetic diet is based on regular food sources and does not require specially prepared foods. Option 1: The foods cannot be consumed freely; the client must still count calories. Option 3: These foods are typically more expensive than regular foods. Option 4: The amounts and types of foods consumed must be considered in planning a diet for clients with diabetes.
NP: Implementation
CN: Physiological integrity
CNS: Basic care and comfort
CL: Application
CA: Adult nursing

25 CORRECT ANSWER: 1
Hypoglycemia occurs in about 50% of clients with Addison's disease. Option 2: Dehydration, a common clinical manifestation of Addison's disease, would cause the BUN level to rise. Option 3: Fluid loss and a decreased serum aldosterone level would result in a lower sodium level. Option 4: Because sodium is substituted for potassium at the renal tubule, serum potassium levels would rise.
NP: Assessment
CN: Physiological integrity
CNS: Physiological adaptation
CL: Analysis
CA: Adult nursing

26 CORRECT ANSWER: 2
High Fowler's position decreases venous return, lowering right ventricular output (preload). Options 1, 3, and 4 all increase venous return and right ventricular output (preload).
NP: Implementation
CN: Physiological integrity
CNS: Reduction of risk potential
CL: Application
CA: Adult nursing

27 CORRECT ANSWER: 3
The client is placed on bed rest to prevent dislodgment of the implant. Visitation restrictions are needed for any client with a radioactive implant because visitors as well as personnel caring for the client may be affected by the radiation. Options 1 and 4: The client's activities must be severely restricted. Option 2: Visitors are restricted.
NP: Implementation
CN: Safe, effective care environment
CNS: Safety and infection control
CL: Application
CA: Adult nursing

28 CORRECT ANSWER: 3
These adverse effects are common when the serum theophylline level is greater than or equal to 20 mcg/ml. The dosage is carefully adjusted according to each client's tolerance and clinical response. Options 1 and 4: None of these is an adverse effect of theophylline. Option 2: Tachypnea is not an adverse effect of theophylline.
NP: Assessment
CN: Physiological integrity
CNS: Pharmacological and parenteral therapies
CL: Application
CA: Adult nursing

29 CORRECT ANSWER: 2
When all team members know what needs to be done, they can work together on the most efficient plan for accomplishing necessary tasks. Delegation can be flexible, ranging from telling a staff member exactly what needs to be done and how to do it to allowing team members some freedom to decide how best to carry out the tasks. Options 1 and 4: These do not allow

for input from team members. Option 3: It is the team leader's job to maintain responsibility for the outcome of a task.
NP: Planning
CN: Safe, effective care environment
CNS: Management of care
CL: Application
CA: Adult nursing

30 Correct answer: 3
According to the history given by the mother, the child's physical problem centers on the ear and the loss of hearing ability. The nodes are most likely due to ear infection or inflammation (otitis media). Option 1: This is possible but not likely, given the history in this case. Option 2: Lymph nodes drain sites of infection proximal to them. Option 4: The nodes in lymphatic cancers, such as Hodgkin's disease, are usually not tender.
NP: Assessment
CN: Physiological integrity
CNS: Physiological adaptation
CL: Analysis
CA: Child nursing

31 Correct answer: 4
The immunization schedule is resumed where it was interrupted; the child should have all deferred 6-month immunizations at this visit. Option 1: This is incomplete; immunization against the Hib virus is now recommended at 2, 4, 6, and 15 months of age. Option 2: There is no need to start the schedule over. A third dose of the live oral poliovirus vaccine is only recommended where polio is endemic; it is not usually given in the United States. Option 3: This is true only if the recommended immunization schedule is followed; however, this client's schedule was interrupted.
NP: Implementation
CN: Health promotion and maintenance
CNS: Prevention and early detection of disease
CL: Application
CA: Child nursing

32 Correct answer: 3
Hand washing and cleaning the perineal area from front to back are the two most important ways to help prevent infection. Option 1: Moist heat does aid healing, but it is not the best way to prevent infection. Option 2: The instructions on cleaning the perineum are too vague; also, the perineal pad should be changed at least four times daily. Option 4: Anesthetic spray will help ease discomfort but does not prevent infection.
NP: Implementation
CN: Health promotion and maintenance
CNS: Growth and development through the life span
CL: Analysis
CA: Maternal-infant nursing

33 Correct answer: 4
This change in color indicates meconium staining, a sign of fetal hypoxia. Options 1, 2, and 3 are all normal during the second stage of labor.
NP: Assessment
CN: Physiological integrity
CNS: Physiological adaptation
CL: Application
CA: Maternal-infant nursing

34 Correct answer: 1
Limit setting is needed to decrease manipulative behavior. A calm, quiet approach may help avoid a power struggle and de-escalate the client's anger. Option 2 is likely to precipitate a power struggle. Option 3 permits the nurse to be manipulated by the client. Option 4 has the potential to antagonize and anger the client.
NP: Implementation
CN: Psychosocial integrity
CNS: Psychosocial adaptation
CL: Application
CA: Mental health nursing

35 Correct answer: 4
The uninterrupted sleep indicates decreased agitation and increased control of the psychotic behavior. Option 1: Ongoing agitated behavior would suggest continuing hallucinations. Option 2: The decrease in blood pressure to subnormal levels could indicate hypotension, a common complication of chlorpromazine therapy. Option 3: Dry mouth and thirst are common adverse effects of chlorpromazine.

NP: Evaluation
CN: Physiological integrity
CNS: Pharmacological and parenteral therapies
CL: Application
CA: Mental health nursing

36 CORRECT ANSWER: 4

Hypoglycemia (insulin shock) is more likely to occur after strenuous exercise. Option 1: The need for insulin decreases with exercise because exercise increases cellular uptake of glucose. Option 2: Food intake would need to be increased before exercise to prevent a hypoglycemic reaction. Option 3: The client is at risk for hypoglycemia, not hyperglycemia.

NP: Implementation
CN: Physiological integrity
CNS: Reduction of risk potential
CL: Application
CA: Child nursing

37 CORRECT ANSWER: 4

Apathy, a sign of depression, indicates that the client may need help in dealing with her feelings about her altered body image. Option 1: Grieving the lost body part is necessary and beneficial to the client's emotional well-being. Option 2: This indicates a healthy ability to incorporate the mastectomy into the client's self-concept and body image. Option 3: This shows her ability to recognize her needs and to take positive steps to meet them.

NP: Evaluation
CN: Psychosocial integrity
CNS: Coping and adaptation
CL: Analysis
CA: Adult nursing

38 CORRECT ANSWER: 3

Adrenalectomy clients must be monitored for signs and symptoms of adrenal crisis, which include severe weakness, nausea and vomiting, and hypotension. Option 1: These are always important data, but they should have been stabilized before the client was transferred from the postanesthesia care unit and are not specific to adrenalectomy. Option 2: These laboratory values may be decreased, but they would not be the focus of the nurse's assessment. Option 4: Serum glucose levels may be monitored, but the nurse's major focus is to check for signs and symptoms of adrenal crisis.

NP: Assessment
CN: Physiological integrity
CNS: Reduction of risk potential
CL: Application
CA: Adult nursing

39 CORRECT ANSWER: 2

Processed foods are usually high in salt. Careful shopping and reading of labels, however, may turn up unsalted varieties of peanut butter. Options 1, 3, and 4: These are all acceptable low-sodium choices; however, eggs may be restricted because of their high cholesterol content.

NP: Planning
CN: Health promotion and maintenance
CNS: Prevention and early detection of disease
CL: Application
CA: Adult nursing

40 CORRECT ANSWER: 2

An output of 30 ml/hour or less suggests inadequate volume replacement. Option 1: This is a large hourly output and would not be anticipated in a postoperative client. Option 3: Normal urine output averages about 50 ml/hour in an adequately hydrated client. Option 4: This indicates fully adequate hydration, possibly beyond what one would expect in a postoperative client.

NP: Assessment
CN: Physiological integrity
CNS: Reduction of risk potential
CL: Application
CA: Adult nursing

41 CORRECT ANSWER: 1

Anorexia is a very early sign of a toxic reaction to digoxin. Option 2: The verbal skills needed for this answer are not reasonably expected in a 1-year-old. Option 3: Digoxin has a diuretic effect because it promotes more efficient cardiac function with subsequent increased blood flow through the kidneys. Option 4: A resting pulse rate of 100 to 120 beats/minute is normal for a 1-year-old.

NP: Implementation
CN: Physiological integrity
CNS: Pharmacological and parenteral therapies
CL: Application
CA: Child nursing

42 Correct answer: 1
Promoting complete compliance with the 10-day course of antibiotic therapy reduces the risk of poststrep rheumatic fever. Option 2: The full course of antibiotics must be taken, even when symptoms are gone. Option 3: Although the mother should not force intake unnecessarily, the child's fever will increase her fluid needs, and some coaxing may be necessary. Option 4: Strep infections are considered contagious for 1 to 2 days after antibiotic treatment is started.
NP: Implementation
CN: Safe, effective care environment
CNS: Management of care
CL: Application
CA: Child nursing

43 Correct answer: 4
Deviation of the uterus to the right indicates that the bladder is full; a distended bladder pushes the uterus up and usually to the side. After the client has emptied her bladder, the involuting uterus should return to the midline. Option 1: This is neither an emergency situation nor one requiring the physician's expertise. Options 2 and 3: Pushing on the uterus or placing the client in a left side-lying position will not resolve the problem, which is caused by a full bladder.
NP: Implementation
CN: Physiological integrity
CNS: Reduction of risk potential
CL: Analysis
CA: Maternal-infant nursing

44 Correct answer: 4
Limit setting is needed to supply ego boundaries and control for clients with borderline personality disorder. Options 1 and 2: These do not impose limits and control. Option 3: This imposes control but does not explain the setting of limits in a therapeutic way.
NP: Implementation
CN: Psychosocial integrity
CNS: Psychosocial adaptation
CL: Application
CA: Mental health nursing

45 Correct answer: 4
The alprazolam relieves anxiety and is also used to manage panic attacks. It has a very low potential for abuse addiction. Options 1, 2, and 3: These antianxiety agents do not work specifically to prevent panic attacks.
NP: Planning
CN: Physiological integrity
CNS: Pharmacological and parenteral therapies
CL: Analysis
CA: Mental health nursing

46 Correct answer: 4
Clients must be told not to try to remove casts themselves. Casts should be removed only by physicians or other trained personnel, usually after X-rays confirm proper alignment of the healing bone. Option 1: The client should not routinely experience extreme pain; if he does, he should report it to his physician. Option 2: The cast should be kept dry. Option 3: Elevating the leg will help prevent edema and pain.
NP: Evaluation
CN: Physiological integrity
CNS: Reduction of risk potential
CL: Application
CA: Adult nursing

47 Correct answer: 2
Gold treatments are used in severe rheumatoid arthritis, not osteoarthritis. Options 1, 3, and 4 show a good understanding of the client's condition.
NP: Assessment
CN: Physiological integrity
CNS: Reduction of risk potential
CL: Analysis
CA: Adult nursing

48 Correct answer: 3
Refined cereals made from corn, oats, rice, or wheat are acceptable foods. Option 1: High-fiber cereals, such as raisin bran, are not al-

lowed on a low-residue diet. Options 2 and 4: Fried foods and highly spiced meats should be avoided.
NP: Implementation
CN: Physiological integrity
CNS: Basic care and comfort
CL: Application
CA: Child nursing

49 CORRECT ANSWER: 3
Coughing and choking result from oral secretions that enter the trachea. The fistula allows secretions to enter the lungs, causing laryngospasm that brings on cyanosis. Option 1: Coarse rales may not be present. Option 2: Choanal atresia, the failure of one side of the nares to open, is unrelated to tracheoesophageal fistula. Option 4: Constipation in a 6-hour-old infant is not assessable.
NP: Assessment
CN: Health promotion and maintenance
CNS: Growth and development through the life span
CL: Analysis
CA: Maternal-infant nursing

50 CORRECT ANSWER: 3
Propantheline bromide is an antispasmodic that works effectively on children. Options 1 and 2: Propantheline bromide is not an antibiotic. Option 4: Propantheline bromide is not a diuretic.
NP: Planning
CN: Physiological integrity
CNS: Pharmacological and parenteral therapies
CL: Application
CA: Child nursing

51 Correct answer: 4
To answer this question correctly, first set up the correct ratio and proportion:

1 mU/minute : 6 ml/hour :: *n* mU/minute : 24 ml/hour

Then multiply the means (6 ml/hour × *n* mU/minute) and the extremes (1 mU/minute × 24 ml/hour). The result is: 6*n* mU/minute = 24 mU/minute. To reduce the equation, divide both sides by 6; the result is *n* = 4 mU/minute. Options 1, 2, and 3 are incorrect calculations.
NP: Implementation
CN: Physiological integrity
CNS: Pharmacological and parenteral therapies
CL: Application
CA: Maternal-infant nursing

52 CORRECT ANSWER: 2
The vibration or thrill felt during palpation ensures that the fistula has the desired turbulent blood flow. Option 1: Pinching the fistula could cause damage. Option 3: Aspirating blood is a needlessly invasive procedure. Option 4: Capillary refill would relay information about perfusion of the extremity but would give no information about the fistula itself.
NP: Assessment
CN: Physiological integrity
CNS: Physiological adaptation
CL: Application
CA: Adult nursing

53 CORRECT ANSWER: 2
Weight gain with truncal obesity, thinning of hair, and purple striae are among the many clinical signs of Cushing's syndrome. Others include hirsutism, menstrual disorders, hypertension, muscle weakness, polydipsia, and polyuria. Option 1: Because these are common signs, notifying the physician is unnecessary. Option 3: The signs are not transient, and calling them insignificant belittles the client's feelings. Option 4: Because of the multiplicity of signs and the resultant changes in body image, the nurse should anticipate mood swings and help allay the client's anxiety by explaining the disease process and plan of care and by allowing ventilation of the client's frustration about her illness.
NP: Implementation
CN: Physiological integrity
CNS: Physiological adaptation
CL: Analysis
CA: Adult nursing

54 CORRECT ANSWER: 4
Although acidosis may result from cardiac arrest, overadministration of sodium bicarbonate can lead to hypernatremic metabolic alkalosis, water overload, and an overall increase in car-

diovascular stress. ABG values are an accurate means of determining blood pH to guide the administration of sodium bicarbonate and avoid alkalosis. Options 1, 2, and 3: ABGs are not used to determine dosages of calcium chloride, epinephrine, or furosemide.
NP: Evaluation
CN: Physiological integrity
CNS: Pharmacological and parenteral therapies
CL: Analysis
CA: Adult nursing

55 CORRECT ANSWER: 1
The client's statement is delusional; delusions are thought content. Option 2: This refers not to content but to how words are put together in thinking and speaking. Options 3 and 4: These refer to other dimensions of assessment.
NP: Assessment
CN: Psychosocial integrity
CNS: Psychosocial adaptation
CL: Analysis
CA: Mental health nursing

56 CORRECT ANSWER: 3
Fatigue is a common complaint among clients receiving radiation therapy, probably due to an increased metabolic rate and the presence of toxic cell breakdown products. Options 1, 2, and 4 are not commonly experienced by clients undergoing radiation therapy.
NP: Planning
CN: Physiological integrity
CNS: Physiological adaptation
CL: Application
CA: Adult nursing

57 CORRECT ANSWER: 3
Exercise has been shown to increase cell sensitivity to insulin. Option 1: While this is important for good health, it is not specific to diabetes. Option 2: The recommended protein intake is 10% to 20% of total calories. Option 4: The frequency of visits will be established by the physician; however, more frequent visits will probably be needed.
NP: Implementation
CN: Health promotion and maintenance
CNS: Prevention and early detection of disease
CL: Application
CA: Adult nursing

58 CORRECT ANSWER: 3
The first step in assessment of this value is to compare it both to the norms for the child's age-group and to her own previous pattern. Option 1: Cardiac problems in this age-group are usually congenital, rarely hereditary. Cardiovascular disease as commonly seen in adults is not manifested in this young age-group. Option 2: Although developmental assessment is always important and delays can be a symptom of cardiac disease or malformation, it is not the first thing the nurse would do in assessing these vital signs. Option 4: Looking for a cardiac defect by ultrasound is a premature step in the assessment process.
NP: Evaluation
CN: Health promotion and maintenance
CNS: Prevention and early detection of disease
CL: Application
CA: Child nursing

59 CORRECT ANSWER: 3
A complete bath is given before the device is inserted. Bathing, especially a complete bath, is usually not permitted during the treatment. Option 1: Nurses are available for short periods or through the intercom. Option 2: A catheter is used to keep the bladder from contacting the radiation source. Option 4: Visitors are restricted during the treatment.
NP: Evaluation
CN: Safe, effective care environment
CNS: Safety and infection control
CL: Application
CA: Adult nursing

60 CORRECT ANSWER: 3
Control over urine elimination during the night commonly does not occur until age $4^1/_2$. Option 1: No evidence exists to indicate infection. Option 2: If the child had not been wetting the bed before hospitalization, she may be exhibiting regressive behavior in response to fears about hospitalization. More information is needed before this can be determined. Option 4: Wetting the bed is not abnormal for a 3-year-old.

NP: Assessment
CN: Health promotion and maintenance
CNS: Growth and development through the life span
CL: Analysis
CA: Child nursing

Selected References

Mental Health Nursing

Boyd, M., and Nihart, M. *Psychiatric Nursing: Contemporary Practice.* Philadelphia: Lippincott-Raven Pubs., 1998.

Johnson, B. *Adaptation and Growth: Psychiatric-Mental Health Nursing*, 4th ed. Philadelphia: Lippincott-Raven Pubs., 1997.

Mental Health and Psychiatric Nursing, 3rd ed. Springhouse Notes Series. Springhouse, Pa.: Springhouse Corp., 1997.

Shives, L. *Basic Concepts of Psychiatric-Mental Health Nursing*, 4th ed. Philadelphia: Lippincott-Raven Pubs., 1998.

Maternal-Infant Nursing

Kenner, C., et al. *Comprehensive Neonatal Nursing: A Physiologic Perspective*, 2nd ed. Philadelphia: W.B. Saunders Co., 1998.

Maternal-Neonatal Nursing, 3rd ed. Springhouse Notes Series. Springhouse, Pa.: Springhouse Corp., 1997.

Nichols, F., and Zwelling, E. *Maternal-Newborn Nursing: Theory and Practice.* Philadelphia: W.B. Saunders Co., 1997.

Child Nursing

Marks, M. *Broadribb's Introductory Pediatric Nursing*, 5th ed. Philadelphia: Lippincott-Raven Pubs., 1998.

Pediatric Nursing, 3rd ed. Springhouse Notes Series. Springhouse, Pa.: Springhouse Corp., 1997.

Wong, D. *Whaley and Wong's Essentials of Pediatric Nursing*, 5th ed. St. Louis: Mosby–Year Book, Inc., 1996.

Adult Nursing

Assessment Made Incredibly Easy. Springhouse, Pa.: Springhouse Corp., 1998.

Black, J., and Matassarin-Jacobs, E. *Medical-Surgical Nursing: Clinical Management for Continuity of Care*, 5th ed. Philadelphia: W.B. Saunders Co., 1997.

deWit, S. *Essentials of Medical-Surgical Nursing*, 4th ed. Philadelphia: W.B. Saunders Co., 1998.

Handbook of Medical-Surgical Nursing, 2nd ed. Springhouse, Pa.: Springhouse Corp., 1998.

Luckmann, J. *Saunder's Manual of Nursing Care.* Philadelphia: W.B. Saunders Co., 1997.

Medical-Surgical Nursing, 3rd ed. Springhouse Notes Series. Springhouse, Pa.: Springhouse Corp., 1997.

Monahan, F., and Neighbors, M. *Medical-Surgical Nursing Foundations for Clinical Practice*, 2nd ed. Philadelphia: W.B. Saunders Co., 1998.

Polaski, A., and Tatro, S. *Luckmann's Core Principles and Practice of Medical-Surgical Nursing.* Philadelphia: W.B. Saunders Company, 1996.

Smeltzer, S., and Bare, B. *Brunner and Suddarth's Textbook of Medical-Surgical Nursing*, 8th ed. Philadelphia: Lippincott-Raven Pubs., 1996.

INDEX

T

U

V

WXYZ